Medical Emergencies at Sea

Medical Emergencies at Sea

A MANUAL FOR THE CRUISING YACHTSMAN

WILLIAM KESSLER, M.D.

Hearst Marine Books *New York*

Library of Congress Catalog Card Number: 85-81990

ISBN: 0-688-04340-2

Printed in the United States of America

First Edition

1 2 3 4 5 6 7 8 9 10

BOOK DESIGN BY JAYE ZIMET

NOTICE

The medical and health procedures contained in this book are based on research and recommendations of responsible medical sources. But because each person is unique, the author and publisher urge the reader, when circumstances permit, to check with a physician before implementing any of them.

The author and publisher disclaim responsibility for any adverse effects or consequences resulting from the suggestions or the use of any of the preparations or procedures contained herein.

CONTENTS

LIST OF ILLUSTRATIONS

Because I am a seagoing surgeon, over the years many sailing friends have asked me for advice prior to setting off on prolonged cruises and circumnavigations. They needed basic knowledge of the medical problems they might encounter. They needed a proper pharmacy; they needed suitable equipment that would not deteriorate in the sometimes damp and moldy environment of a boat at sea. Most of all, they needed relief from the understandable anxiety that accompanied their lack of medical knowledge. I have been distressed by the absence of a comprehensive medical guide specifically geared to yachtsmen, as well as by the inadequacy of most seagoing first-aid kits. It seems totally incongruous to me that a proper yacht will set off with the most sophisticated navigational equipment and a bare minimum of equipment for medical emergencies.

The essence of safety at sea is an awareness of the strength of the elements, of wind and water. The wise yachtsman takes on these forces only to the extent that he and his vessel can handle them, and uses them to his best advantage. These forces are overpowering and the winner (or loser) in any head-to-head confrontation is entirely predictable. Thus the prevention of injuries at sea lies in a healthy respect for these forces, an ego that is attuned to reality, a boat that is seaworthy, and an ability to predict the boat's reactions.

The very forces that drive a boat through the water can create equally strong adverse effects. Sheets under tension can tear out an eye. Objects not fastened down become missiles. Sharp corners become weapons. Wet, slick decks become skating rinks and the absence of safety harnesses and lifelines leads to death by drowning. Boating should be a pleasurable, safe recreation, and this book deals with the accidents that can undermine that pleasure. It is designed to provide serious yachtsmen with comprehensive, up-to-date information so that they can approach medical problems with some logic as well as with some ability to judge the seriousness of many injuries.

Readers will learn to recognize specific medical emergencies they can treat, what symptoms are part of the natural course of a particular injury, and finally, what is beyond the scope of the average yachtsman, that is, when to seek professional help and how soon. This book not only gives hands-on advice in the event of injuries and medical emergencies but provides information for judging the seriousness of certain injuries and their potential for permanent harm. It also describes the contents of the ideal medical kit and life-saving techniques that should be learned before setting out to sea. Healthy sailing!

CHAPTER 1

The Skin

As the largest organ in the body, and because it is exposed to the external world, the skin is most vulnerable to injury. The skin has the unique ability to regenerate when part of its thickness is damaged or lost. We all know that a scrape (abrasion) or a superficial burn (blister or sunburn) will heal. But when full-thickness skin is injured or lost, it will not regenerate and heals by the formation of dense scar tissue. This process takes longer than regeneration and is dependent on the area of loss and on whether there is secondary infection.

BURNS

SUNBURN

Underestimating the intensity of the sun in tropical latitudes, coupled with prolonged exposure to both direct and reflected sunlight, makes this a common, painful, and sometimes disabling injury. Often forgotten is the fact that one can sustain an extremely severe sunburn while snorkeling, which involves lying on one's belly admiring the beauty of the coral world below while the neck, back, arms, and legs fry in the light-gathering aquamarine waters of the tropics. Lotions and creams are washed off, leaving exposed skin *totally unprotected.*

Treatment

Since most sunburns are first degree (redness) or second degree (blisters, partial thickness), therapy must be aimed at making the victim more comfortable, preventing further injury, and combating the systemic effects of the burn if they are present. Aspirin or Tylenol should be used for pain relief. Various balms, lotions, and creams are available commercially, and those containing aloe (or the use of natural aloe which grows in most tropical climates) seem to be most helpful.

A weak tannic-acid solution such as weak tea is comforting. So are cool, wet sheets. Another kitchen remedy is water and cornstarch, applied as a thick paste. Antibiotic ointments should be avoided in the primary care of sunburn. Liberal amounts of fluids by mouth should be encouraged to prevent and counter dehydration.

Prevention

Simplicity itself. *Cover thy skin.* This should not be beyond anyone's capabilities. Bimini tops on yachts are a help. (But remember the reflected sunlight!) The newer blocking agents containing PABA (para-aminobenzoic acid) in alcohol (5%) are most effective and now come numbered as to the effectiveness of their ultraviolet filtration, with "15" providing 15 times, or "8" providing 8 times, an individual's natural protection. These should be applied *before* exposure and be reapplied after swimming or excessive sweating. They should not be allowed to come in contact with the eyes. Although "15" is called a "total" blocker, this is misleading, for a fair-skinned blond will still burn. Therefore, wide-brimmed hats, kerchiefs, long-sleeved shirts, pajamas, and thin turtlenecks for snorkeling, especially *early* during intense exposure, are all essential.

ROPE BURNS

The palms of the hands are extremely thick, as are the soles of the feet. Thus deep burns are rare, but superficial burns occur frequently. The best therapy is prevention, that is, gloves and a healthy respect for the power of the wind and sails. You should also work on toughening the skin of your palms.

Treatment

The aim is to prevent further wound contamination, alleviate pain, and provide a suitable environment for healing. The affected areas should be thoroughly cleansed. An antibiotic ointment such as Neosporin should be applied and covered by nonadherent gauze and a bulky dressing. Change the dressing daily until the burn is healed.

FIRE AND GALLEY-STOVE BURNS

Accidental burns produce a variety of injuries depending on their extent, location, and depth. Explosive burns are frequently associated with respiratory burns as well as corneal burns. Explosive burns are also associated with "burn shock," which may preclude treatment of the burn wound itself until it is controlled. For the yachtsman, evaluation of the extent and depth of the burn is of importance: Any partial-thickness burn that involves more than 15 percent of the body surface should be treated in a medical facility, as should a full-thickness burn.

Evaluate the extent of burns by the Rule of Nines: The surface of the body is divided into regions that represent 9 percent or a multiple of 9 percent. (See illustration 1.)

Estimating Burn Depth

The history of the burn provides a clue here. Scalds usually produce partial-thickness burns. When clothing is afire,

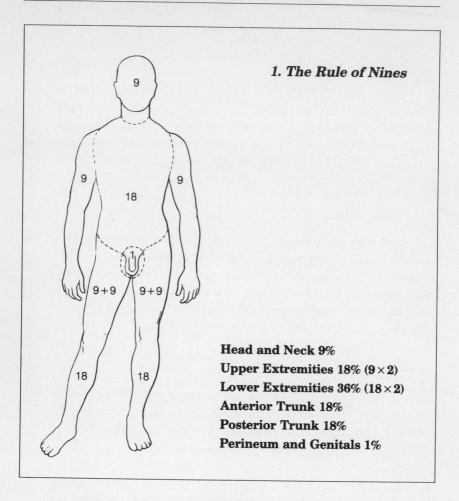

1. The Rule of Nines

Head and Neck 9%
Upper Extremities 18% (9×2)
Lower Extremities 36% (18×2)
Anterior Trunk 18%
Posterior Trunk 18%
Perineum and Genitals 1%

the burns are usually deeper. Flash-fire burns *may be* superficial.

Treatment

Extensive burns, that is, partial-thickness burns of greater than 15 percent, or deep dermal burns, should be evacuated to a medical facility. So should serious burns involving hands, feet, or genitalia and burns associated with other major trauma and inhalation burns. Treatment of shock and respiratory support is usually essential early in an exten-

First degree burns (partial thickness)	redness
Second degree burns (partial thickness)	blister formation painful sensation to air movement
Third degree burns (full thickness)	charring or white (pale skin) anesthetic to pinprick no pressure blanching appear dry

sive burn. Intravenous crystalloid (saline or Ringer's solution) should be started if rapid air evacuation is not possible and may be lifesaving. In the treatment of severe burns, immediate lifesaving measures involve attention to the following (in order of importance):

Alleviate airway distress: Factors that hint at airway burns are:

1. Facial burns
2. Singeing of eyebrows and nasal hair
3. Carbon particles in the nose or mouth
4. Black (carbonaceous) sputum
5. A history of unconsciousness or confusion coupled with confinement in a burning environment.

The above findings suggest airway burns. Respiratory support (endotracheal tube) will be needed.

Stop the burning process by removal of burning clothing or chemically saturated clothing.

Provide an intravenous line for circulatory support.

Therapy for Minor Burns

Minor burns may realistically be treated aboard. The aim of therapy is to prevent contamination and infection by gently cleansing the burn wound to remove dirt, debris, and loose skin. Blisters should be left intact. They form a good dressing. Bacteria can be reduced by using dilute iodine preparations, for example, one-half-strength Betadine. A mixture of household bleach diluted 1:60 (1 quart to 15 *gallons* of water) is an effective antibacterial solution. Protective dressings should then be applied. Impregnated gauze, fluffed 4×4 gauze sponges, and Kurlex or Kling roller-gauze splints may be fashioned. These dressings should be changed every third day, at minimum. If infection is apparent, saltwater soaks and antibacterial ointments (Silvadene, Neosporin) may be used.

It is important to realize that a deep second-degree burn may be converted to a full-thickness burn by infection. Burns that involve an arm or leg on all sides are special and should be professionally handled even if they do not cover an extensive area.

WOUNDS

Superficial Wounds

These are common wounds that heal well and rapidly by regeneration. Therapy is directed toward avoiding infection by copious irrigation and by removal of any foreign material imbedded in the skin to avoid tattooing as well as infection. This may involve mechanically scrubbing the wound. These wounds may be treated "open" or "closed." The open method allows a surface crust to form. The closed method provides an artificial crust by using gauze (Adaptic), which may or may not be impregnated with antibacterial agents. Care must be taken to prevent infection under the scab, and if infection is suspected, saline soaks (1 tablespoon salt per quart of water) at room temperature repeated four times daily for 15 minutes will usually suffice to clear the infection and promote healing.

Deep Wounds

At the very least, these wounds involve the full thickness of the skin, that is, subdermal fat is visible in the depths of the wound, and may involve important structures beneath the skin—major blood vessels, muscles, tendons or nerves. It is important to keep in mind that the basic aim of our body's biologic systems is preservation. Given a basically healthy person whose metabolism is functioning normally, all the elements necessary for repair are present, and little else is needed to help the body help itself. Healing may be retarded, however, by both external and internal factors. External factors such as cold and hunger may sap the energy needed for fighting infection. Internal factors include the extent of the injury and the presence of pain and anxiety, as well as blood loss.

Evaluation of a deep wound involves determining if underlying structures are involved. Nerves are either sensory or motor, so that motion beyond the wound (away from the body) and sensation beyond the wound are tests of their involvement. Possible bone fractures may be evaluated by testing the stability of the part or by visual evidence of a broken bone with lacerations of the forearm. Hand and finger tendon function can be evaluated by flexing and extending the fingers.

This initial evaluation is to determine if professional medical care is needed. The two instances where this conclusion would be drawn involve major arterial injury and an open fracture where bone fragments are exposed to the environment.

Major Arterial Injury

Such injuries are fortunately uncommon. Each finger and toe has two arteries supplying it. There are two major arteries at the wrist and ankle. Generally, sacrifice of one of these paired vessels does not involve tissue loss. The most serious arterial injuries involve the femoral artery at the groin, the popliteal artery behind the knee, the brachial artery in the upper arm (axillary artery) and the carotid arteries in the neck. Injury to these arteries (open injury) is accompanied by impressively brisk bright red bleeding, pulsing and forceful and frightening to all involved. If the artery is cut crosswise (illustration 2), the ends usually constrict and even major hemorrhage will slow down or stop (illustration 3).

However, if the vessel is torn laterally on one side, hemorrhage usually continues at a brisk pace. This is frequently the case in penetrating wounds (illustration 4).

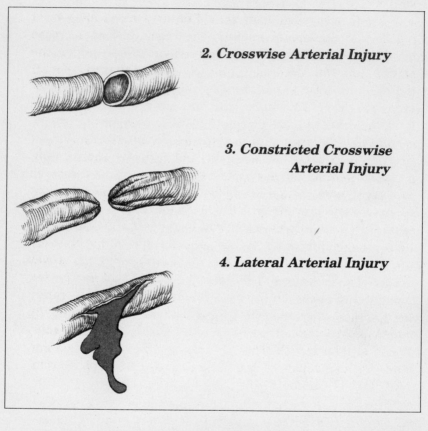

2. Crosswise Arterial Injury

3. Constricted Crosswise Arterial Injury

4. Lateral Arterial Injury

Control of hemorrhage, with almost no exceptions, can be achieved by *elevation* of the part and *direct pressure* over the bleeding site. This can be accomplished by holding a thick compress over the wound. The tendency is to release this pressure frequently to "peek" at the wound and see if bleeding has been controlled. *Don't do it!* Hold pressure for ten minutes *by the clock,* without a peek. And if after ten minutes, the bleeding is still profuse, repeat for another ten minutes. A roller bandage, such as an Ace, can be helpful in keeping even pressure on the wound. Care should be taken to make certain that this wrap is not so tight that circulation is further impeded. Blueness (cyanosis) of the fingers or toes or nail beds is a clue to poor circulation beyond the pressure wrap.

The use of tourniquets should be condemned for several reasons. If improperly applied, they may in fact increase bleeding by shutting off only the venous outflow and not the arterial inflow to the area. If properly applied they also cut off the collateral flow to the extremity from other arteries, leading to gangrene. Tourniquet pressure can also damage underlying nerves. A tourniquet is not a substitute for a compression dressing. Its use should be reserved for those *rare* instances where an adequate and correctly applied compression dressing and elevation fail. In such cases, it may be lifesaving, even though it may doom the limb to amputation. In an effort to prevent limb loss from tourniquet gangrene, a regulation was in force during the early part of World War II that a tourniquet must be released for five minutes every thirty minutes. This regulation was abandoned when it was realized that lives were being lost from the blood loss for ten minutes each hour. In my experience, a tourniquet is rarely needed, and the decision to use one is made simple by *massive, uncontrollable* loss of blood. The blind use of clamps should also be decried. They can damage nerves severely and may preclude repair of the lacerated blood vessel by compounding its trauma.

Open Fractures

Do not attempt to push exposed bone ends back beneath the skin. Simply cover the wound with a sterile dressing and splint. (See Chapter 3: Musculoskeletal Injuries.)

Cleansing the Wound

"Dilution is the solution to pollution!" Thorough washing of the wound with copious amount of salt solution (preferably sterile) is the simplest and most effective method of cleansing a wound. Boiled and cooled seawater is fine. Boiled and cooled water with one tablespoon of salt per quart is fine. Unsterile seawater would be the next choice. Pulsating irrigation, as with a Water Pik or manual bulb syringe, is an excellent method of washing a wound. Mechanical spray bottles (some now have jet nozzle adjustments) will work as well. They should be thoroughly cleansed before use and irrigated with boiled water. The key to irrigation is volume. Irrigate, reirrigate and re-reirrigate. Then start again! Soap and water can be used on the normal skin around a wound. As a final application, dilute Betadine is ideal. Clorox diluted 1:60 (1 quart to 15 gallons of water) is effective as well. A brush may be needed for mechanical debridement (removal of dead tissue and foreign matter), and a surgical scrub brush impregnated with Betadine or pHisoHex is ideal. (See The "Ideal" Medical Kit.) Peroxide (3%) is also a good irrigant and I have found it useful for controlling oozing from capillaries, probably due to its bubbling action, which greatly increases exposed surface area.

Closing the Wound

No wound *has* to be closed. Many wounds *should not be* closed. Suturing, if done improperly, complicates the healing of wounds and sets the stage for infection. Furthermore, repairing the scar on a wound poorly or improperly sutured is more difficult than repairing one on an unsutured wound. But any scar can be repaired, if necessary.

The desire to "make things right" after a lacerating wound is overpowering and primitive. Some aboriginal tribes went so far as to use pincer ants with little lobsterlike claws that were applied to the edges of an open wound. The pincers would shut, closing the wound, and then the bodies would be broken off, leaving the pincers as clamps until the wound was either healed or infected—probably the latter.

The concept of "delayed" wound closure has been a surgical precept for decades and is a basic tenet of military wound care.[1] Following initial cleansing and debridement, these wounds are *not* closed but lined with fine mesh gauze, lightly packed with fluffed-up gauze sponges, covered with an outer dressing and splinted if necessary. Delayed primary closure is then done three to eight days later. The infection rate is very low, and the ultimate cosmetic results are good.

For practical purposes, no wound has to be closed immediately except a hole in a major blood vessel or a wound that exposes the brain or its linings. Facial wounds that expose bone or cartilage should be cleansed and covered, and antibiotic ointment and nonadherent gauze (Adaptic) applied. Definitive treatment can be delayed for days. Closure of the superficial layers of any deep wound leaves a "dead space" below, which fills with blood or serum and forms a perfect medium for the growth of bacteria. Infection then makes the initial wound even more extensive, increases the "morbidity" of the wound, and may do irreparable damage.

The message of this section on "closure" is thus: *Leave wounds open!!* Cleanse them. Protect them from further injury and contamination by adequate *dry* dressings. Use antibiotics on the wound. Control pain if it is severe and let nature and eventually a physician do the rest. If indeed a superficial laceration lends itself to closure, use Steristrips or butterflies. (See illustration 5.)

A few words about the scalp. Scalp lacerations bleed profusely because of the very rich blood supply in the area. This can be frightening. Pressure again is the key to stopping the bleeding.

Coral Cuts

These razorlike cuts from the exoskeleton of coral frequently become infected. Treatment should include thorough scrubbing with soap and water and a scrub brush to remove embedded pieces of coral. Hydrogen peroxide may be used, fol-

[1] *Medical Surgical Practice of the U.S. Army in Viet Nam,* Year Book Medical Publishers, Nov. 1966.

lowed by alcohol and an antibiotic powder (tetracycline, Neosporin powder).

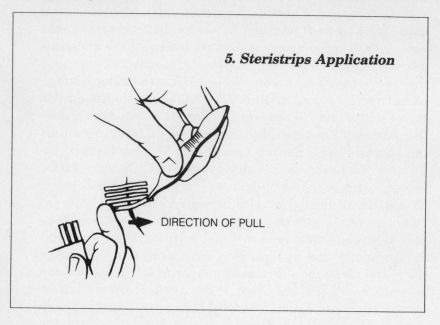

5. Steristrips Application

DIRECTION OF PULL

MISCELLANEOUS

INSECT BITES

Stinging Insects

Statistically, death is a rare event from the bites or stings of such insects as bees, wasps, and ants (the Hymenoptera) and one has a fivefold *greater* risk of being struck by lightning! However, an understanding of the basis of the irritation caused by these creatures will alleviate not only anxiety but pain. The venom glands of stinging insects are normally located astern, in their tails, and the venom itself contains a histamine-releasing component, which generally causes most of the symptoms in man. Most stings require no treatment. However, overwhelming attacks by swarms of hundreds of thousands of bees (such as the "killer bees" of Brazil) can cause death.

Anaphylaxis, a serious hypersensitivity reaction, is the usual cause of death from stings, and the honeybee is the major culprit. Anaphylaxis is a reaction to venom caused by an aberrant antigen-antibody response, a sensitivity reaction, the mechanism for which is triggered by the sting but not caused by the venom itself. The reaction is systemic rather than local. If one is known to be hypersensitive, desensitization should be done, generally by an allergist, prior to exploring areas with few medical facilities.

Anaphylaxis is a catastrophic allergic situation. Early recognition of symptoms is the basis for successful therapy. The triad of an itchy rash, "tightness" in the throat, difficult breathing or collapse is diagnostic of this reaction, when coupled with a bite or sting or the administration of a drug. The itchiness may occur by itself or be associated with respiratory distress or profoundly low blood pressure. Wheezing may or may not be present. The hypotension may lead to sudden loss of consciousness. The hallmark treatment is epinephrine. It may be given:

1. Into the injection site (the sting) (0.3 ml of a 1:1,000 solution = 300 mg) or
2. Subcutaneously into a nonoccluded extremity (0.5 ml of 1:1,000 solution = 500 mg) or
3. If the victim is in cardiovascular collapse, it can be given intramuscularly or preferably intravenously. The intravenous dosage is either 0.1 mg (1 cc of 1:10,000 or .1 cc of 1:1,000) or 1 mg may be added to 500 cc of normal saline if an I.V. is running.
4. It can also be injected into the vascular network under the tongue if an open vein is not available.
5. A final route is via the endotracheal tube if one is placed and no I.V. is available. Give 0.5–1.0 mg directly into the endotracheal tube.

The placement of a tourniquet above the sting site is controversial. If symptoms are not fullblown this may work. However, if symptoms are classic, it probably will not help and, as previously described, may be harmful.

Treatment should also be aimed at enhancing oxygenation by giving oxygen by mask or endotracheal tube with assisted breathing ("bagging"). Aminophylline, 500 mg diluted in 250 ml of I.V. solution, should be given if wheezing (bronchospasm) is evident. This solution should be given over *one hour*.

Treatment of hypotension (decreased blood pressure) should include cortisone (hydrocortisone sodium succinate), 100 mg given intravenously either direct or diluted in an I.V. levarterenol bitartrate (Levophed), 4 ml of a 0.2% solution added to 1,000 ml of I.V. solution given at a rate of 2 ml/ minute, has been suggested.

Late reactions (longer than 1 to 15 minutes) can be treated with the antihistamine Benadryl (diphenhydramine), 50 mg orally.

Itchy reaction alone requires similar therapy. Treatment of the local reaction, which is not an allergic reaction but a direct effect of the venom, consists of elevation, cool compresses, analgesics, and Benadryl if severe. Antibiotics are not indicated since the venom itself kills bacteria. Anyone who has a known history of such a hypersensitivity would be well advised to carry or have immediately available an "allergy" kit. These are commercially available (Epi Pen Labs, Port Washington, New York, or ANA-Kit, Hollister Stier, Spokane, Washington) or can be made up. Basically they consist of epinephrine (1:1,000) and a hypodermic.

Other Insects

Mosquitos, gnats, and fleas produce mainly local effects with pain, itching, swelling, and redness, and treatment is symptomatic. Papaya (Adolph's meat tenderizer) applied as a paste, or baking soda paste, seems to be soothing, especially if applied right away. Benadryl (25–50 mg) helps the itching.

Use antibiotics only for secondary infection. Prevention is a lot easier than the inconvenience caused by these pests.

BOILS AND CARBUNCLES

Of the multitude of bacterial infections of the skin, boils (furuncles) and carbuncles are the most frequent. They represent infections of the hair follicles in the skin, usually staphylococcal in origin. A boil is an infection of one hair follicle, while a carbuncle is an infection of several adjacent hair follicles that drains through multiple openings. Some of the causes are thought to be poor skin hygiene, diabetes, local skin trauma with chafing and the introduction of bacteria, or certain dietary factors (high fat, high carbohydrate) yet to be proven. Treatment should include hot soaks with salt water or boric-acid solution and opening and drainage when "ripe." Penicillin given orally or intramuscularly for two to four days will help. If boils become recurrent, hexachloraphene soap (Dial) should be used daily, and any focus of infection (teeth, tonsils, urinary tract) should be ruled out. Extended tetracycline therapy has helped chronic cases.

HIVES

Caused by a release of histamine from specific body cells, these lesions (urticaria) are commonly caused by a hypersensitivity (allergic) reaction. Reactions to drugs (especially penicillin), food (especially seafood, strawberries, nuts, milk products), insect bites and stings (see above), physical agents such as the sun, infections, and some internal diseases all have been implicated as causative agents in the production of hives. Treatment—systemically with oral Benadryl (25–50 mg) and locally for the itching—is usually sufficient. A myriad of home remedies exists for hives. A starch or oatmeal bath helps (1 cup for a shallow tub), and a 1% camphor solution in alcohol, applied locally, relieves the itch. This is rarely an emergency at sea—unless the rash is the warning signal for an anaphylactic reaction.

CHAPTER 2

Venomous and Toxic Marine Animals

These ye shall eat of all that are in the waters: all that have fins and scales shall ye eat: and whatsoever hath not fins and scales ye may not eat; It is unclean unto you.
Deuteronomy 14: 9–10, circa 1400 B.C.

Never eat a fish that blows itself up like a balloon.
Survival on Land and Sea,
U.S. Navy, Office of Naval Intelligence, 1944

These words of advice, separated by thousands of years, hold true today, for in general, poisonous fish have bony spines that are covered with venom. Some are encased in a boxlike frame and some have naked skin without spines or scales.[1]

In order to simplify the medical aspects of poisonous and venomous marine animals, this chapter will be divided into sections involving marine animals that sting, those that have *venomous or dangerous spines,* and those that are *poisonous to eat.*

STINGING ANIMALS

These animals, that is, jellyfish, sea anemones, corals, and *hydra,* have complex stinging apparatuses. They all have tentacles that contain stingers called nematocysts, and they

[1] D. I. Macht, "An Experimental Appreciation of Leviticus XI 9–12 and Deuteronomy XIU 9–10," *Hebrew Medical Journal* 2:165–170

all appear symmetrical anatomically. The stingers inject toxin into the skin on contact, and this toxin may be very potent. Symptoms increase with the amount of toxin injected, which in turn is a direct manifestation of the amount of contact with the skin. These species are present in salt water in temperate zones, but the most severe reactions seem to occur in subtropical or tropical zones. The Portuguese man-of-war, one of the most common of the jellyfish, have air bladders, usually brightly colored, and long tentacles. With their air bladders full, they blow with the wind along the sea surface and many of them tend to occur together, like an armada; hence their name. The most toxic of the jellyfish is the *sea wasp*, common in Pacific waters, capable of causing death in seconds.

Contact with the more toxic species is followed by intense pain, usually burning in nature. Raised purplish weals or welts appear on the skin along lines of contact and these may blister. Contact with less toxic species may cause "prickling" sensations or itching. There may or may not be generalized symptoms and these may be rapid or delayed. They include cramps and muscle spasms, severe throbbing headache, numbness of extremities, nausea, chest pain, difficulty in swallowing, and shocklike states. Death is rare but has been reported. Massive skin contact with less toxic species can cause severe reactions.

Treatment

Since the nematocysts remain toxic as long as they are in contact with the skin, any adherent tentacles should be removed at once, using protective gloves, or with the hand wrapped in cloth, towels, even seaweed. The involved areas should be washed with cool seawater, followed by dilute household ammonia, vinegar, or alcohol. Coalescing or adherent tentacles can be removed by sprinkling on flour, baking soda, or baking powder and scraping the resulting paste with a dull knife, cardboard, plastic, etc. Rerinse the areas with similar solutions (dilute ammonia, baking-soda solution or vinegar, gasoline or shaving lather followed by shaving). Steroid cream (cortisone, Kenalog) should be applied to decrease the inflammation and anithistamines should be given orally (Benadryl 25–50 mg, Pyrabenzamine 25–50 mg) and continued every four hours as necessary. If generalized symptoms are severe, calcium gluconate (10 cc of a 10% solution), preferably injected intravenously, slowly over five minutes, will relieve muscle spasm. Treatment for shock or respiratory depression may be necessary.[2,3] Papain, the enzyme in the papaya plant, may have a beneficial effect in detoxifying the nematocysts and relieving the stinging. Application of Adolph's meat tenderizer has the same effect. Application of adhesive tape or Scotch tape may help to remove the nematocysts.

Sea wasps, the most toxic of jellyfish, indigenous in Pacific waters from Japan to Australia, may require tourniquets—again at the risk of limb loss. Antivenin is available (Sea Wasp Antivenene, Department of Health, Commonwealth Serum Laboratories, Melbourne, Victoria, Australia) and cruising yachtsmen spending time in these waters may be well advised to have this aboard.

Note: Do *not* put fresh water on neumatocysts that adhere to the skin. Also do not *rub or scratch* the areas. These stimuli tend to cause the "firing" of the undischarged nematocysts.

ANIMALS WITH SPINES

These marine animals produce poisoning or wounds by puncturing the skin. They include many different species such as sea urchins, stingrays, stonefish, scorpion fish, catfish, some segmented worms, and cone shells. These species are

[2]South Cott, "Tropical Jellyfish and Other Marine Stingings," *Military Medicine,* 124 (8) 569–79, 1959.
[3]M. B. Strauss, "Injuries to Divers by Marine Animals: A Simplified Approach to Recognition and Management," *Medicine* 139:129, 1974.

usually nonaggressive and many are hard to see among rocks and in sand. They may be stepped on accidentally (stingrays, sea urchins) or may be taunted into attacking by inquisitive divers (stonefish, scorpion fish)—although the stonefish is so ugly and menacing, it's hard to imagine taunting it. The **sea urchin,** a relative of the starfish, is abundant in tropical waters. It has many black spines, which it uses to "walk." Although a specific toxin has not been identified with these spines, they can produce intense pain when they puncture the skin. Rarely, generalized symptoms can occur (lightheadedness, dizziness, numbness of lips, and weakness of limbs). Treatment involves removal of the spines mechanically, as one would remove a splinter. Oil or grease (suntan oil, for example) may help in this job. Thorough cleansing of the area followed by local use of antibiotics or antiseptics (Betadine) will help prevent secondary infection.

Stingrays have a whiplike tail with a serrated stinger at its base. They are bottom dwellers, and injury is produced when the fish is accidentally stepped on. It then uses its tail offensively. Penetration of the skin causes intense pain from the venom, and generalized symptoms (cramps, sweating, vomiting, abdominal pain, drop in blood pressure) may occur. (Death has been reported when chest or abdomen has been penetrated, but this is rare.) Treatment consists of cleansing the wound by irrigation and removing foreign material. The injured area should be soaked in *hot, hot* water, as hot as can be tolerated. The toxin is destroyed by heat. Relief of pain is usually instantaneous. This treatment should continue for thirty to sixty minutes, adding hot water intermittently to keep the water as hot as tolerable. Care should be taken to avoid blistering or scalding the skin. After this period, the wound can be thoroughly cleansed. Administration of antihistamines and analgesics may be indicated to control inflammation and pain. These wounds may become infected. Antibiotics should be used selectively.

Stonefish (Synanceja) are ugly rock dwellers that have a row of highly venomous stinger spines along their backs, usually thirteen in number. (Unlucky?)

Scorpion fish (Scorpaenidae) similarly produce injury by their dorsal stingers. According to Halstead,[4] injury is usually caused by careless handling or by stepping on the dorsal stingers of a partially buried fish. Some scorpion fish are aggressive and will attack if a hand reaches within striking distance of their spines. Dead fish can also be injurious when improperly handled (see Halstead). These fish also have anal and pelvic stingers. Punctures usually cause excruciating pain. The area around the wound may become bluish (cyanotic), and the area may be hypersensitive, tingling, hot and swollen. Blisters may form. Severe and potent poisoning may cause respiratory distress and circulatory collapse. Death may occur rapidly. Secondary wound complications are common, with tissue loss and gangrene. The affected limb may become paralyzed for a while. Gastrointestinal symptoms are sometimes seen.

Treatment involves cleansing the wound to prevent further infection, and control of pain by immersion of the affected part in *hot, hot* water (as with stingray injuries). Antitetanus measures should be taken. Analgesics (morphine or Demerol) may be necessary for severe pain. An antivenin is available and is provided by Commonwealth Serum Laboratories in Melbourne, Australia. It is recommended that an initial dose of 2 milliliters be given intramuscularly or intravenously, followed by a second dose if symptoms persist. An injection of emetine hydrochloride into the site of the sting may relieve the pain, as will a few drops of 1:1,000 solution of potassium permanganate (see S. Weiner, "Stone Fish Sting and Its Treatment," *Medical Journal of Australia* 2:219–222, 1958).

The effects of the venom on the cardiovascular system may be life threatening and circulatory support may require hospitalization after the initial treatment for shock (see page 89). Stings by **weaver fish** inhabiting the Eastern Atlantic and Mediterranean coasts, **toadfish,** and **surgeonfish** should

[4] Bruce W. Halstead, *Dangerous Marine Animals,* 2d ed., Cornell Maritime Press, 1980. Used by permission of Dr. Halstead, Director, International Biotoxicological Center, World Life Research Institute, Colton, California.

be treated in the same manner as those from stonefish.

Sea snakes (sea vipers, sea serpents) inhabit the Pacific and Indian oceans, ranging widely from Africa and Japan to India and Australia. They are docile, shallow-water reptiles, carnivorous and venomous. Poisonings (see Halstead) usually occur while handling nets or wading and accidentally stepping on the snake. Characteristically, the bites are initially *painless,* the victim not being sure of what has happened. The fang marks are tiny, multiple punctures. Hours later, generalized symptoms occur in serious bites: muscle pain, stiffness, progressing to generalized muscular weakness and paralysis, ascending from the legs upward. Difficult breathing and facial paralysis may follow. Collapse may then occur with dark urine (myoglobinuria). Muscular movements are painful, if possible. Treatment is a true emergency since absorption is rapid. It is estimated that only 25 percent of sea-snake bites result in poisoning. Halstead stresses the importance of establishing a diagnosis before therapy by the following criteria:

1. History of opportunity for contact
2. A painless bite
3. Presence of fang marks
4. Positive identification of the snake
5. Development of symptoms

Recommended treatment includes *putting the part and the patient at rest.* Keep the part lowered. A tourniquet should be applied one joint above the bite and tightened enough to cut off venous and lymphatic circulation but not arterial circulation. It should be loosened for *ninety seconds every ten minutes.* It should not be applied at all if the bite is over thirty minutes old, and it should not be continued for more than four hours.

Antivenin should be administered intravenously after testing for sensitivity to horse serum (see package insert). Adrenalin should be available to counteract sensitivity to the horse serum. Halstead recommends the use of a polyvalent antivenin that includes a *krait fraction* if sea-snake antivenin is unavailable and injecting it intramuscularly at a site distant from the bite. (Sea-snake antivenin is available from Commonwealth Serum Laboratories, Melbourne, Australia, and Venin Research Laboratories, Penang, Malaya.) Support of the kidneys by maintaining blood pressure and alkalinization of urine, as well as respiratory support, may be necessary. (Corticosteroids are equally useful to prevent the generalized effects of the toxin.)

POISONOUS FISH

SHELLFISH POISONING

Paralytic shellfish poisoning, PSP, is common in many tropical areas following ingestion of bivalve, filter-feeding shellfish such as oysters, clams, and mussels. Saxitoxin, the specific toxin, is extremely powerful and is reported to be fifty times stronger than curare. The toxin paralyzes the muscles and is present in plantlike one-celled organisms called dinoflagellates. During periods of heavy infestation with these organisms, the water is actually discolored (red tide, red water) by this "bloom" of dinoflagellates. Not only are the shellfish highly toxic, but mass mortality of fish ensues and can be a serious commercial and public-health nuisance.

Ingestion of toxic shellfish is followed by onset of symptoms, either rapidly (thirty minutes) or delayed (twelve hours). Numbness and tingling first occurs in the mouth and lips and then spreads to the extremities. There may be unsteadiness and inability to stand or walk. Gastrointestinal symptoms such as vomiting are common. In severe cases, respiratory distress may follow and may lead to death within the first twelve hours. Survival after this period is associated with a good prognosis.

Treatment should be aimed at reducing the amount of ingested toxin by induction of vomiting and/or by gastric lavage, if possible, followed by supportive therapy. Valium (diazepam) may reduce anxiety. Adequate fluid intake can help the kidneys to excrete the toxin, and respiratory support may become necessary.

SCAMBROID POISONING

This poisoning is caused by ingestion of inadequately preserved fish. Scambroid fish are generally dark-meated, migratory fish including mackerel, skipjack, tuna, and bonito. The poisoning is thought to be due to an infestation of these fish with bacteria, especially the *Proteus* species that metabolize histidine to histamine. Large quantities of histamine and another similar amine (saurine) accumulate rapidly (four hours) in these fish. Clinically, the symptoms of scambroid poisoning are similar to histamine intoxication and cause intense headache, flushing, dizziness, asthmalike symptoms with shortness of breath and wheezing, palpatations, changes in blood pressure, abdominal cramps, nausea, vomiting, and diarrhea. There is generalized weakness and a characteristic metallic taste in the mouth. Symptoms vary with the amount ingested. Mild reactions can be treated with antihistamines (Benadryl 50 mg, Pyrabenzamine). Severe reactions should be treated with epinephrine hydrochloride: 0.1 to 0.5 ml of a 1:1,000 aqueous solution given subcutaneously. Scambroid intoxication can be prevented by eating susceptible fish only when absolutely fresh or promptly refrigerated. If there is the slightest hint of spoilage, the fish should be discarded. Any dark-meat fish that has a "peppery" or sharp taste should not be eaten.

CIGUATERA

Cigueratoxic fish are too numerous to list, almost too numerous to count. Reportedly, some four hundred species are involved in this serious and sometimes fatal poisoning. The toxin is present in reef fish of a wide variety, and generally involves shallow-dwelling or bottom-dwelling, nonmigratory fish living in tropical island environments. Their toxicity is due to algae (*Gambierdiscus toxicus*), most likely associated with a brown seaweed they ingest. These fish are usually territorial, so the reef fish in one area may be toxic while the same species in another area may be safe to eat. The fish themselves do not appear ill, but transmit the toxin to carnivorous fish or to man. The larger the fish, the more toxic they are. (See illustration 6.)

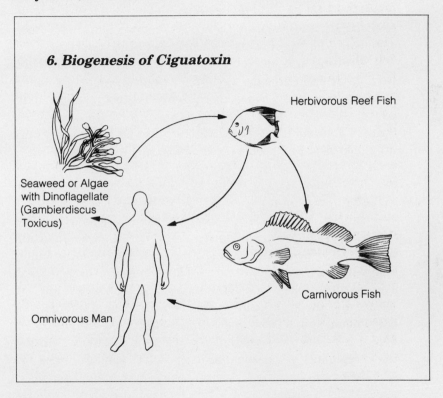

6. Biogenesis of Ciguatoxin

Herbivorous Reef Fish

Seaweed or Algae
with Dinoflagellate
(Gambierdiscus
Toxicus)

Carnivorous Fish

Omnivorous Man

The onset of symptoms varies from almost immediately to twenty-four hours, but usually within six hours. The initial symptoms may be gastrointestinal (nausea, vomiting, abdominal pain with diarrhea) or neurologic with numbness and tingling about the mouth and lips, dizziness, progressive weakness, and exhaustion. An unusual "heaviness" of the muscles is described as well as "electricitylike" shooting pains in the extremities. There is also altered sensation from hot and cold objects. Neurologic symptoms may persist for months. Symptoms appear to be directly related to the amount of fish eaten, and fatalities have been reported.

Treatment is aimed toward eliminating the poison from the body (by induction of vomiting or by gastric lavage, if possible) and combating the effects of the poison. Give atropine sulfate, calcium gluconate (10 cc of a 10 percent aqueous solution), Demerol for pain if necessary, and oxygen and respiratory support if needed. Since the toxin has not been chemically identified, there is no known antitoxin.

Prevention is based on the natural history of the illness. Do not eat large predatory reef fish such as snapper, grouper, jack, or barracuda. Since moray eels are notoriously toxic, never eat tropical eels. Try to catch fish in open water rather than in lagoons or on reefs. Eat only small portions of any unknown fish, and seek native advice about local reef fish.

PUFFER FISH

Puffer fish (blowfish, porcupine fish, spikefish, etc.) are found in the Indo-Pacific, Japan, Hawaii, the tropical Atlantic, West and South Africa, the Florida Keys, the West Indies and Bermuda (generally warm seas). They are highly toxic. The specific toxin, tetrodotoxin, has been isolated and its effects are known. It blocks the transmission of impulses in both motor and sensory nerves and affects skeletal and cardiac muscle (see Halstead). These fish are most toxic during their reproductive seasons, and the skin, gonads, intestine, and liver appear to be the most toxic parts. Fugu (Japanese puffer fish) is a delicacy in Japan. Special statutes require fugu cooks to become licensed and the fish is prepared according to carefully prescribed methods (see Halstead) and generally served raw, as sashimi. Numerous poisonings have occurred from the ingestion of testes, livers, and intestine of these fish and according to Halstead, the taste of the fish is not its only attraction. It seems that the attenuated poison still present in the fish as prepared has an exhilarating effect and produces a euphoric "high."

Symptoms of puffer-fish poisoning develop within the

first hour. Paresthesia—a tingling sensation about the mouth, lips, tongue, extremities, fingers, and toes—occurs commonly and may progress to numbness. Profuse sweating, salivation, chest pain, tachycardia, and extreme weakness are followed by respiratory distress and paralysis involving first the muscles of the throat and larynx and then the extremities. The victim becomes completely paralyzed but remains conscious until death. Skin manifestations are redness and swelling, tiny punctate hemorrhages in the skin, followed by blistering and peeling of the involved skin. Halstead reports two victims who were left for dead, but who became conscious and recovered, one, seven days later. Death usually results from respiratory paralysis and occurs within six to twenty-four hours. The death rate approaches 50 percent (see Halstead).

Treatment is, again, directed at the symptoms. There is no specific antitoxin. To rid the body of ingested poison, induced vomiting, emetics, large quantities of sodium bicarbonate, apomorphine, laxatives, and enemas have been recommended. Respiratory stimulants such as caffeine and Coramine may be helpful. Intravenous fluids, Metrozol, and artificial respiration should be used if necessary to prolong life. Lobeline and epinephrine have questionable value.

Prevention: Don't eat puffer fish.

CHAPTER 3

Musculoskeletal Injuries

FRACTURES AND DISLOCATIONS

A **fracture** is a break in a bone. A "chip" is a fracture. A "crack" is a fracture. Any injury that acutely changes the stability of a bone is, by definition, a fracture. A fracture can be *simple,* that is, a crack without displacement of bone fragments, or *complex,* with displacement, multiple fragments, and severe associated injuries to nearby muscles, nerves, joints, blood vessels, and tendons. If a fracture is associated with penetration of the skin it is called a *compound* or *open* fracture. (See illustration 7.)

When a bone is broken, the ends of the fragments of tissue around the fracture site bleed, causing pain and swelling. This can be made more severe by movement of the bone fragments and "rough handling." The pain starts about five to twenty minutes after the fracture occurs, and the swelling usually increases for the first twenty-four hours. Rapid swelling indicates more severe hemorrhage.

Dislocations are derangements of joints and always involve injury to the ligaments, the "standing rigging" of the body, which holds the bony structure of the body in place. They may also involve fractures and are associated with hemorrhage into the joints, which causes pain as well as limitation of motion.

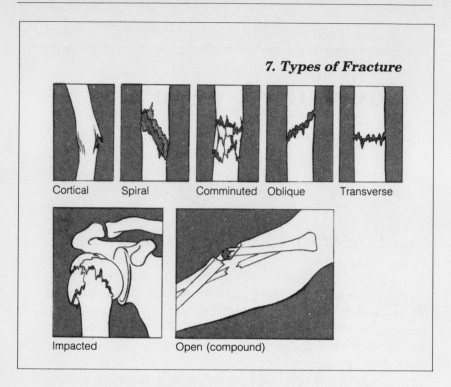

7. Types of Fracture

Cortical   Spiral   Comminuted   Oblique   Transverse

Impacted   Open (compound)

Initial Evaluation

Generally, and with few exceptions, fractures and dislocations are not life threatening. (Exceptions are fracture of the cervical spine with cord injury, depressed fracture of the skull, bilateral rib fractures with a "flail" (unstable) segment, or massive pelvic fractures with internal hemorrhage.) They do, as mentioned, bleed, and in some fractures the blood loss can be massive. It is estimated that femoral (thighbone) fractures can lose 800 to 1400 cc of blood (1 to 3 pints). Pelvic fractures can bleed even more profusely, and shock, necessitating blood replacement, can occur. Multiple injuries or multiple fractures compound the situation so that life-threatening conditions should be evaluated and treated first: that is, respiratory and circulatory problems. Following this initial assessment, the musculoskeletal injury can be evaluated.

Fractures are frequently associated with nerve or blood-vessel injury and the assessment of sensation, pulse, and motion beyond the fracture site is important.

General Principles of Fracture Treatment

"Splint 'em where they lie." Consider all musculoskeletal injuries as fractures. Immobilize the patient until the diagnosis can be made. Be gentle, and refrain from manipulation of the injured part more than is essential to comfort. Be attentive to the status of the circulation beyond the fracture site. Don't compromise it by binding the extremity too tightly. Make the splint fit the patient rather than the other way around. If the fracture is open, wash and dress the wound with sterile dressings before applying a splint. *Do not attempt to push exposed bone ends back in.* Adequate splinting involves the immobilization of the joint above and the joint below the fracture. Do not attempt to straighten a dislocation unless there is evidence of poor circulation to the part beyond the injury. (See page 21.)

At sea, with cramped quarters and constant motion, musculoskeletal injuries involving *weight-bearing* bones (legs and spine) take on a different priority from injuries involving *non-weight-bearing* bones. The availability of medical treatment, or of medical advice via radio-telephone, and the availability of evacuation facilities (a Coast-Guard helicopter, for example) must be considered in the case of these injuries. The comfort and transportation of a patient with weight-bearing-bone injury is obviously more complicated to achieve. Even the straightforward act of moving the patient from topside to below or vice versa becomes much more complicated if the patient cannot bear weight after splinting, and the burden on the entire crew is much greater. Therefore, efforts should be made to provide medical treatment promptly for those so injured. Evacuation of open fractures is an urgent priority. Antibiotics should be started if a delay will be more than six hours.

Splinting

Before moving the injured person, absolute immobilization of the injured part is essential, and involves forethought and organization. There is usually no hurry, so *don't be in a hurry*. For injuries involving the lower extremity above the knee, the use of a long padded splint from base of toes to armpit or the use of the opposite limb, with padding between the legs, is effective and facilitates transportation. (See illustration 8.)

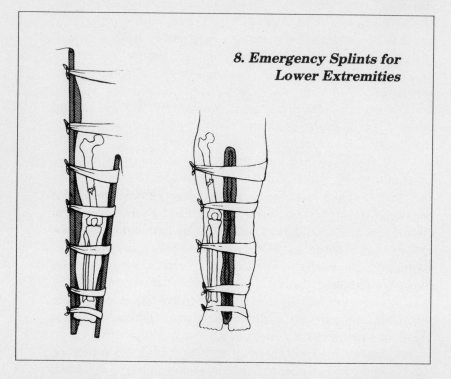

8. Emergency Splints for Lower Extremities

Adequate padding is essential and it should conform to the patient. Small bunk pillows or blankets are fine for fractures of the lower extremity from the knee down. Air splints are very useful and should be part of the medical kit. They must be used with some caution, however, to avoid overinflation or underinflation. They are available in full-leg, half-leg, full-arm and half-arm conformations, with or without zipper. The zippered type is easier to apply and involves less movement of the injured part. They should not be used for injuries above the elbow or above the knee. If they are left on for long periods, peeling of the skin can occur. (See illustration 9.)

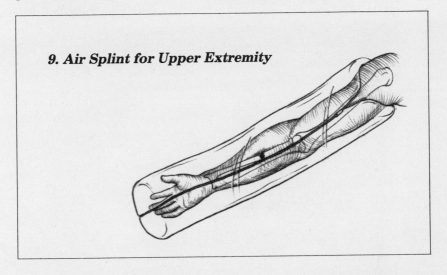

9. Air Splint for Upper Extremity

A little practice with these splints on normal extremities will give a feel for the proper inflation. Frequent checks of circulation and immobilization will help. Remember that hot air expands and compression can change as temperature fluctuates. Finger pressure should just indent the properly inflated air splint.

If air splints are not available, injuries from the knees down may be splinted with rigid splints such as a padded board, heavy cardboard, sail batten, etc.

In either case, when the splint is applied, fore and aft traction may be necessary to lift the extremity or to maintain position while the splint is being placed *under* or *alongside* the break. The extremity should be grasped above and below the fracture and *gentle* traction applied, slowly and steadily. The extremity is moved *as a unit* and as little as possible. The person holding the extremity must maintain this unit until the splint is positioned *by a second person*. (See illustration 10.)

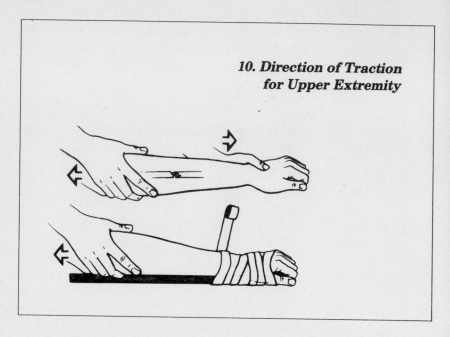

10. Direction of Traction for Upper Extremity

For injuries above the elbow, a sling and swathe provide proper immobilization. (See illustration 11.)

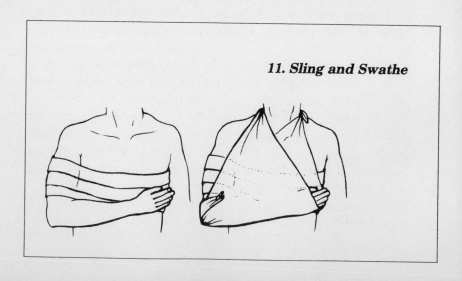

11. Sling and Swathe

Fingers and toes are best splinted by taping securely but not constrictively to the adjacent finger(s) or toe(s). Padded wooden sticks can be used for fingers as well.

The ankle can be well splinted with a pillow if air splints are not available.

SPECIFIC PROBLEMS

FACIAL FRACTURES

Usually, the majority of facial fractures are not life threatening. The initial approach should be:

1. Establish an adequate airway, either an oral airway or by *cricothyroidotomy* (see p. 132). This may be necessary in fractures of the mandible (jawbone) or if the injury involves a facial "crush"—the so-called "pumpkin face syndrome." In these situations an oral airway will be inadequate.
2. Control hemorrhage *by direct pressure.*
3. Control shock and evaluate any *other injuries.*

THE SPINE

Immobilize all potential spine injuries on a long board (door, etc.) with pillows or sand-filled bags on either side of the head. Move the patient *as a unit.* Spine injuries are urgent priority for evacuation to a medical facility.

THE CLAVICLE (COLLARBONE)

A low-priority fracture. Analgesics for pain are indicated. Healing will occur with no treatment. A figure of eight dressing does more for the "treator" than the "treatee." (See illustration 12.)

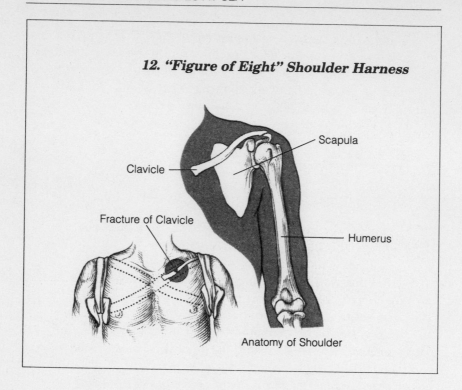

12. *"Figure of Eight" Shoulder Harness*

Scapula

Clavicle

Fracture of Clavicle

Humerus

Anatomy of Shoulder

THE SHOULDER

For an incomplete dislocation, use a sling and swathe.

With a *complete dislocation* of the shoulder joint, reduction is sometimes very difficult, especially in a strong young male. In many instances the dislocation is recurrent and will spontaneously slip back into position. The vast majority of these injuries will be dislocated toward the front of the body (anterior dislocations), and they are sometimes associated with fractures and nerve injury. Check for signs of neurological involvement, such as loss of sensation or motion in the hand.

If no medical help is available, reduction should be attempted. (See illustration 13.) The diagnosis is difficult in a heavily muscled individual, but there is an appreciable depression below the very tip of the shoulder, and pain is experienced if the elbow is forced inward.

13. Anterior Dislocation of Shoulder

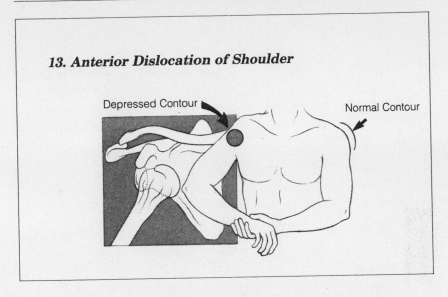

Depressed Contour   Normal Contour

Reduction is potentially dangerous and can cause damage to the structure about the shoulder joint. The safest method is by *traction* and demands cooperation and *relaxation* on the part of the injured person. Analgesics (Demerol) will help. Excessive force should not be used nor any manipulation other than straight-line traction at a 45-degree angle to the body. (See illustration 14.)

The patient lies flat on his back. The wrist is grasped and gentle traction is exerted at 45 degrees *without any lateral motion*. Reduction is accompanied by an appreciable "give" of the arm as the humerus slips into position and the deformity disappears. This procedure should not aggravate the pain. A sling and swathe should then be applied and X rays taken when possible. If this technique fails after a one to two minute attempt, it should be abandoned and the injured person transferred to a medical facility.

Alternative methods involve the use of weight suspended from the wrist (not grasped), either with the patient on his abdomen and the weight hanging straight down or over a chair back. (See illustration 15.)

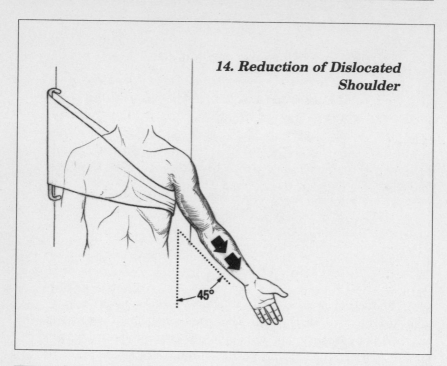

14. Reduction of Dislocated Shoulder

45°

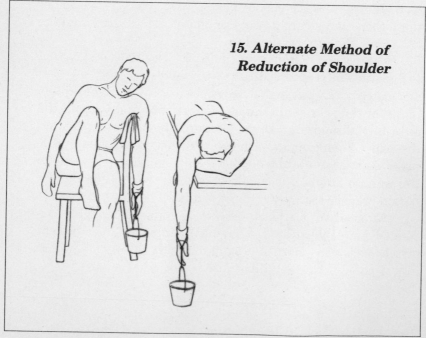

15. Alternate Method of Reduction of Shoulder

THE HUMERUS

Most upper-arm fractures are adequately treated by a sling and swathe. Fractures in the middle third of the bone may cause injury to the radial nerve. Such an injury can be identified by the occurrence of "wrist drop" or the inability to extend the wrist. Swelling, discoloration (ecchymosis), and distortion of the upper arm are common because of the hemorrhage associated with these fractures.

THE ELBOW

Dislocation is usually caused by a fall upon the forearm and is frequently accompanied by fractures and circulatory insufficiency to the hand, as well as injury to the ulnar and median nerves. These are serious injuries and need prompt reduction. Serious disability can result from improperly handled elbow injuries and medical advice should be sought. Many such fracture-dislocations require surgery, and neglected fractures are associated with serious complications including gangrene of the forearm.

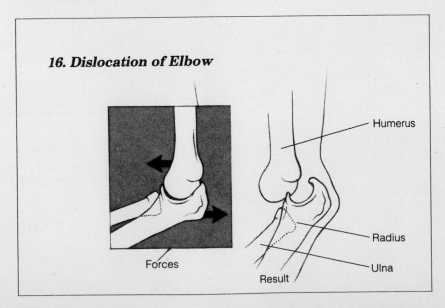

16. Dislocation of Elbow

Humerus

Radius

Ulna

Forces

Result

For these reasons, fractures and fracture-dislocations of the elbow are urgent priority factures. Medical therapy should be sought and delay in therapy is to be avoided. *Avoid constricting circular wraps about the elbow.* Splinting should be without constriction. Delayed blood vessel and nerve complications (Volkmann's contracture) are not unusual with severe elbow injuries (See illustration 16.)

THE FOREARM

Fractures of *both bones* of the forearm are unstable, and even under the best of conditions, surgical reduction may be necessary. The fracture is usually quite apparent because of the angulation of the forearm that accompanies it. Emergency treatment should be aimed at adequate splinting, using gentle in-line traction and immobilizing both the wrist and the elbow. (See illustration 18.) The full-arm air splint is ideal for this. Severely angulated fractures should be straightened by gentle traction, in line with the axis of the arm, before the splint is applied.

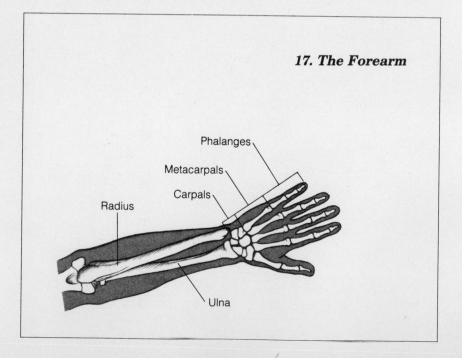

17. The Forearm

Phalanges

Metacarpals

Carpals

Radius

Ulna

Fractures of *either the ulna or the radius* are more stable, since the one intact bone acts as a strut, maintaining length. Healing may be slow. Since the bones of the forearm rotate about one another, splinting should involve the elbow as well as the wrist to reduce rotation. These fractures are second-priority fractures and delay in medical help can usually be tolerated without serious consequences.

THE WRIST

The most common fracture of the wrist involves the very ends of the ulna and radius (Colles's fracture). Injury is usually caused by a fall on an outstretched hand, which has been extended to stop the fall or protect the rest of the body. The resultant displacement of the bone ends may cause "silver-fork" deformity. Impaction (one fragment being driven into another, resulting in shortening) is common in these fractures, as is comminution (multiple fragmentation).

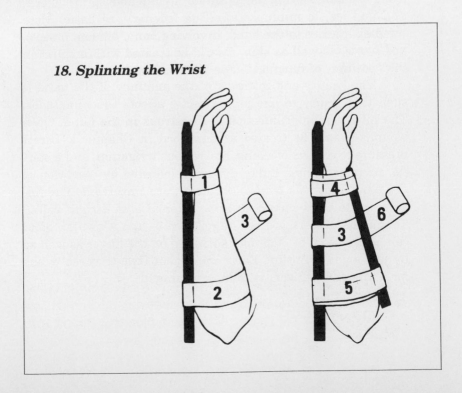

18. Splinting the Wrist

Splinting of the Hand and Fingers

Since most cruising yachts do not have X-ray equipment, it will be anyone's guess whether a fracture is present or not unless there is obvious angulation. Splinting of the hand and fingers takes on a primary therapeutic role at sea, therefore, and the technique is herewith described.

The "position of function" of the hand and fingers is seen in illustration 20. It is the position the hand naturally takes at rest. It is "cupped" as if the hand were covering a tennis ball. It is in this position that the hand should be dressed and immobilized. The dressing of the hand consists of several layers. The first layer, if there is a wound, should be nonadherent gauze (Adaptic, etc.). This is followed by fluffed-up gauze sponges to provide bulk and compression. These fluffs are used to "fill the cup" of the palm and fingers. Individual pieces of gauze "flats" (nonfluffed) can be placed between the fingers. The thumb forms the diameter of the hemisphere (cup) and the tip of the thumb is almost touching the index fingertip. (See illustration 21.)

20. The "Position of Function"

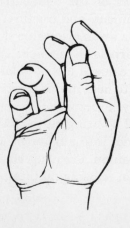

Elasticized cotton bandage (Kling, Con-Form) is then wrapped around the entire hand, exposing only the tips of the fingers so that circulation can be checked at will. *The bandaged hand should be elevated.* Fingers are best splinted in the same position. Malleable finger splints (Alumifoam) can· be cut and shaped individually. Take care not to wrap too tightly. The splint, to be effective, should extend up the wrist. (See illustration ·21.)

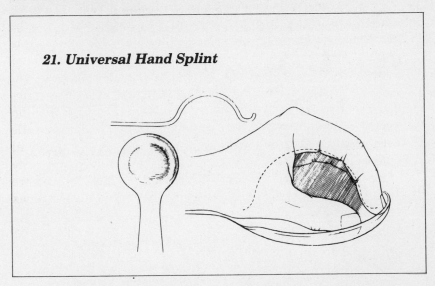

21. Universal Hand Splint

A "universal" hand splint is available and is an excellent addition to the medical kit (Rajowalt). Properly padded, it keeps the hand and wrist in the "safe" position and can be used for either hand. It also can be reused and comes in small, medium, and large.

THE RIBS

Probably the most common fractures aboard are due to being thrown into a stationary object in surging or heavy seas. Rib fractures are painful but rarely serious. Analgesics for pain are necessary, especially for sleep. Strapping may help but can impair respiration. Bilateral rib fractures may have serious respiratory complications. Underlying lung damage is unusual except in chest injuries involving great force. X ray is indicated when available. These are low-priority fractures.

THE PELVIS

Fractures of the pelvis are rarely isolated and are generally associated with blunt abdominal trauma. These fractures will be discussed in Chapter VI: The Abdomen.

THE LOWER EXTREMITIES

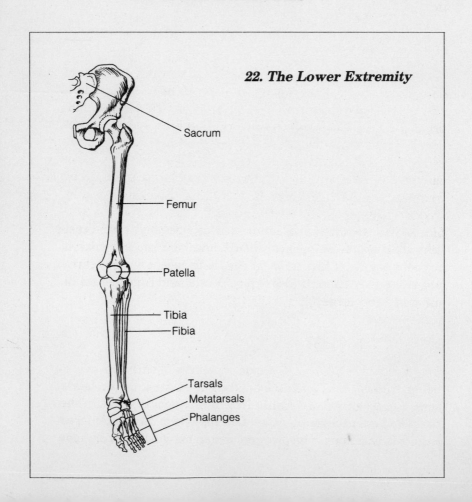

22. The Lower Extremity

Sacrum

Femur

Patella

Tibia
Fibia

Tarsals
Metatarsals
Phalanges

The Femur (Thighbone)

These fractures characteristically bleed profusely into the tissue of the thigh. Two to three liters of blood loss is not uncommon. The powerful muscles of the thigh also tend to cause overriding and shortening of the bone. These fractures should be splinted as shown in illustration 8 and medical attention sought. As previously stated, the burden of an immobile cruise mate who cannot bear weight is to be considered in respect to the confines of the yacht and the effect on the entire crew. Give plenty of fluids to counter blood loss. Hospitalization with traction is frequently necessary.

The Knee

These injuries are particularly dangerous because of damage to the popliteal artery and nerve. Reduction is difficult and usually involves skeletal traction. These are high-priority fractures. Dislocation of the knee involves tremendous force and is always associated with disruption of the ligaments and capsule of the knee joint. The knee can dislocate in any direction, and dislocation may be complicated by fractures associated with it. Reduction of this dislocation by traction should be done immediately, especially if there is blood-vessel involvement. This is usually done with the knee flexed if the dislocation is posterior, that is, if the lower leg is behind the knee. Straight in-line traction would be used if the lower leg is in front of the knee. The knee should then be splinted and medical advice sought for X rays and further therapy.

The Lower Leg

Fractures of the fibular shaft alone, except at the ankle joint, are usually not serious, although they are painful. The head of the fibula by the knee (outer aspect) may be injured and its proximity to the *peroneal* nerve may cause neurologic damage, which involves "foot drop" (inability to lift up or extend the toes), as well as insensitivity to pinprick over the top of the foot and outside of the ankle. This type of injury requires precise reduction of fragments to prevent permanent nerve injury. Fractures of the upper sides of both bones of the lower leg (tibia and fibula) may involve the knee joint. These fractures should be splinted and medical help sought. Lower down, in the shaft of these bones, as with both bones of the forearm, instability is characteristic. These fractures as well should be splinted and medical help sought.

The Ankle

These fractures are caused either by rotary motion or by forced motion of the leg with the foot fixed. The ligaments of the ankle joint tend to prevent this type of motion, which is a partial dislocation, and injury to these ligaments is always associated with ankle fractures. A "sprain" of the ankle is the overstretching of these ligaments. Fractures occur when the ligaments "give way." Frequently, with sprains of the ankle, a snapping or "pop" is heard or felt and is not necessarily an indication of a fracture. Splint and X-ray when available. Delay in therapy is acceptable if unavoidable, but keep the ankle elevated and do not bear weight on it.

The Heelbone

These fractures are caused by falls from heights. Ignored, they can cause long disability. Splinting, elevation, and medical therapy are helpful for these second-priority fractures.

The Toes

These are usually dealt with by treating the symptoms. Alleviate pain, minimize swelling, splint if the toe is painful. If the toe is askew, in-line traction and taping to the adjacent toe is acceptable treatment and may be all that is needed.

*   *   *

In summary, fractures of the leg will be more difficult to manage aboard. Fractures of the arm, except for the elbow, are second-priority fractures, except if nerve or blood-vessel damage is associated with them. The time-honored principles of ice, elevation, pain relief, and adequate splinting are hallmarks of fracture management at sea. Open fractures are high priority, as are serious knee fractures or fracture dislocations, and elbow fractures. The importance of splinting and gentle handling is stressed.

CHAPTER 4

Head Injuries,
Spine Injuries

For our purposes, the *skull* must be considered as a bony box containing evolution's greatest gift, the human brain. The skull is tough; the brain is delicate. The danger of a fractured skull is directly related to its effect on the underlying brain tissue and its blood vessels. If there is no underlying damage, the head injury, even one involving a fracture of the skull, is insignificant.

A blow to the skull, if transmitted to the brain, is more serious. A "concussion" is essentially a "shock" to the brain. It manifests itself by an alteration in consciousness or awareness or memory or any other brain function.

Aside from the master-control function of the brain cells, there are two other characteristics that are important in considering head injuries. First, the brain tissue has many blood vessels. Second, the brain tissue needs oxygen to survive. Every system in the body is geared to provide oxygen to brain tissue. Armed with this information, we can understand the following essentials of caring for head injuries:

- Anything that impairs the oxygen supply to the brain is lethal to it. Assuring an adequate airway is essential.
- Since the brain is encased in a rigid bony box (the skull), any swelling of the brain can be transmitted only *inward* to the brain tissue itself. Essentially, swollen brain tissue becomes crushed against the unyielding skull.

limited space of the cranial cavity, displacing vital brain tissue.

The *dura* is a membrane that covers the brain. Following head injuries, blood can collect, forming a hematoma, either outside the dura (extradural) or inside the dura (subdural). **Extradural hemorrhage** is frequently associated with a fracture of the skull that lacerates a major arterial vessel, (the middle meningeal artery), or a large vein. In the typical case, a blow to the head is sustained above and slightly forward of the ear. There may be a period of unconsciousness after which the injured person regains consciousness and seems quite "lucid" for a variable period of the time (minutes to hours). He may complain of headaches during this "lucid interval" and gradually not only does the headache become worse, but the level of consciousness diminishes, and vomiting, elevated blood pressure, and slowing of the pulse occurs, pointing to increasing intracranial pressure. The pupil on the side of the blow may become enlarged (dilated). One can clearly see the need for keeping records of the patient's level of consciousness, pulse, and blood pressure during the early hours following a head injury. In most cases, the clinical course is not "typical" and the "lucid interval" may not be as apparent as described.

Extradural hematoma is a first-priority injury. The blood must be removed and the bleeding controlled, preferably before the patient becomes comatose. This is done by drilling holes in the skull (burr holes). Every effort must be made to air-evacuate those so injured to a medical facility. The death rate is high.

Subdural hematoma usually involves rapid bleeding from vessels associated with a laceration of the brain substance. There is extensive brain damage and the outlook is usually poor. These patients usually do not have the so called "lucid interval" unless the bleeding is a very slow, venous ooze. The development of symptoms thus may take days or weeks (chronic subdural hematoma) and patients with even trivial head injuries, especially older people, where there has been brain shrinkage associated with age, may develop confusion or a convulsion weeks after the injury. These patients generally respond well to removal of the clot, as opposed to patients with acute arterial bleeding (acute subdural hematoma).

It should be obvious that anyone who has a depressed skull fracture, an open skull fracture, or a blow to the head followed by decreasing levels of consciousness, development of a dilated pupil, paralysis, decreasing pulse rate, and increasing blood pressure needs medical care as soon as possible. These injuries have high mortality rates and should not be managed aboard if humanly possible. A concussion or contusion, followed by *steadily improving signs,* may be managed aboard.

SPINAL-CORD INJURIES

Nowhere is the initial approach to the patient as critical to the eventual outcome as in spinal injuries. Any inappropriate movement of an unstable spine may cause irreversible damage to the spinal cord and permanent paralysis.

For practical purposes, the spinal column can be looked at as a stack of dominoes, one atop the other. Imagine that these dominoes, end on end, are held together by straps running up and down their edges, allowing flexibility yet maintaining alignment. Running along with these dominoes is the spinal cord, which contains the myriad of "wires" that connect the circuitry of the brain to the machinery of our muscles and extremities, as well as the cables that carry sensation impulses to our brains. Any break or dislocation can threaten these vital motor and sensory bundles of "wires." The dominoes themselves, if forcibly flexed or extended, can impinge on this cable, interrupting the circuitry.

With this concept in mind, it becomes apparent that the maintenance of alignment is essential in any injury of the spine.

THE CERVICAL SPINE

That portion of the spine extending from the base of the skull through the neck to the level of the upper chest is called the cervical spine. This portion of the spine is particularly vulnerable when a blow to the head from a fall transmits force upward, as with a dive into shallow water. Symptoms of injury in most instances are: **pain,** localized to the back of the neck, **limitation of motion,** and **spasm of the neck muscles.**

The initial survey of such an injured person should involve evaluation of sensory and motor function of the extremities and torso. Ask if the injured person has any alteration of sensation in any extremity. Can he move fingers and toes? Arms and legs? Do they feel strange? Are they weak? Can they feel touch and pinprick? Can the person feel if a toe is moved upward (extended) or downward (flexed)? This initial neurologic assessment is very important, as is reassessment at regular intervals. For patients with immediate paralysis following a cervical spine (and cord) injury, the prognosis is very poor. For those with function, even if altered, prognosis is much better.

As mentioned earlier in relation to splinting techniques, any motion of the neck should be avoided. If the patient is on his back, sandbags, pillows, or a neck roll to fill the gap between the patient's neck and the deck should be used. The patient should be moved *as a unit*. Gentle head traction in the long axis of the body will keep the neck from flexing or extending. If the patient is lying facedown, he should be "logrolled" onto a long board (which can't be done without several people to help) and supported as a unit on the board, with straps and support at the sides of the neck.

A "Philadelphia" collar, which is a rigid plastic collar whose separate halves attach with Velcro straps, allowing the front half of the neck to be examined if necessary, is the most practical method of immobilizing the cervical spine. It is virtually indestructable. Short of this, a stiff collar, towels, pillows, or sandbags can be effectively used as a cervical collar or splint. The patient should be *transported on his back,* never sitting, and on some type of flat rigid board such as an old door, a raft, even the bottom of a flat-bottomed dinghy, necessity being the mother of invention. As a matter of course, all head injuries should be considered to involve cervical-spine injuries until proved otherwise, and the transportation of all spinal injuries, cervical, thoracic, lumbar (see below), should be the same.

If a diving accident occurs—a frequent cause of cervical-spine injury—and the victim is approached in the water, it is just as important to support the head and neck as one unit. If the patient is facedown in the water, an arm should be passed under the head toward the chest. The other arm "sandwiches" the head and chest for support and is kept that way until the patient is turned faceup, as a unit. Following this, extrication from the water can be accomplished by sliding an appropriate flat surface under the patient, floating it to shore and removing it while holding the patient stable. Mouth-to-mouth can be done if necessary at any time.

THE THORACIC SPINE

The twelve thoracic vertebrae (those in the upper back) and the ribs form the thoracic cage. Sprain, dislocation, or fracture are relatively uncommon injuries here except in high-speed accidents or in falls from heights, and are usually of a compression type (the collapse of one domino). If there is no spinal-cord injury, these can be treated by bed rest and eventually a back brace. The same can be said generally for the *lumbar spine,* the lower back. If no nerve damage exists, bed rest and eventual X rays, braces, etc., can be used. If there is nerve damage, surgical reduction (laminectomy, fusion) may be necessary, and thus these are higher-priority injuries.

CHAPTER 5

The Chest

CHEST TRAUMA

For our purposes we will define chest trauma as injuries sustained to the "lower" airway, that is, from the Adam's apple (larynx) to the lung tissue, or to the bony chest cage itself. We have already discussed injuries to the thoracic spine and uncomplicated rib fractures. To understand the anatomy of the chest, it is simplest to conceive of the chest as a closed system (a vacuum) in which the lungs are suspended. (See illustration 23.) The stoppered bottle is *rigid but expandable,* and tends to return passively to its original shape. The space between the balloonlike lungs and the inside lining of the chest is the pleural cavity. This normally has a negative pressure and does not communicate with the atmosphere. (See illustration 23.)

The lungs, however, *do* communicate with the atmosphere through the "lower" and "upper" airways. It is obvious that anything, from the teeth on down, that *obstructs* the free flow of oxygen-containing air will interfere with the exchange of carbon dioxide for oxygen through the capillaries of the lungs. Anything that *mechanically* interferes with the expansion of the chest, or expansion of the lungs, does essentially the same thing. Also, anything that *fills the pleural space* (for example, blood or fluid) or *changes the pressure* from normal negative to positive will inhibit expansion of the lungs and the *gas exchange.*

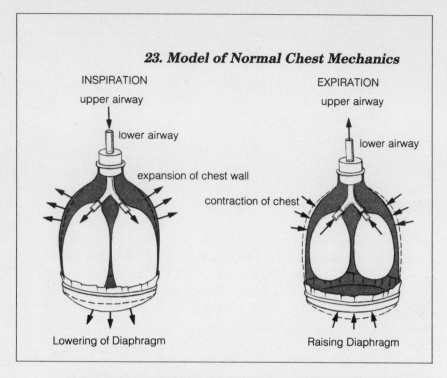

23. Model of Normal Chest Mechanics

INSPIRATION
upper airway

lower airway

expansion of chest wall

Lowering of Diaphragm

EXPIRATION
upper airway

lower airway

contraction of chest

Raising Diaphragm

Because of these physical characteristics—a semirigid chest wall containing air-filled lungs—there are clues that help establish a diagnosis quickly. Physical examination is important in chest injuries and involves four steps.

Look. Watch the injured person breathe. Does the chest wall move normally up and out on inhaling? Down and in on exhaling? Do both sides move? Are there bruises or wounds? Are the veins in the neck distended or bulging? Is the windpipe in the middle of the neck? Is the victim blue (cyanotic)? Gasping? Is breathing "labored"?

Feel. Feel the chest. Is there tenderness? Is there a grating sensation, indicating a broken bone? Is there any abnormal motion (instability) of the chest wall?

Listen. Listen to the chest (with or without a stethoscope). Here again, a few minutes of practice on a normal person helps. The normal passage of air in and out of the lungs produces audible, characteristic sounds. Anything that interferes with this exchange of air during breathing will alter the normal sounds or produce characteristic sounds that are abnormal, such as snoring, wheezing, gasping. Are breath sounds present? On each side? Are they both the same in quality? In loudness? Is there any crackling or bubbling (rales)? Are there rattling noises (ronchi)? Remember, a stethoscope can also be used for *engine and pump noises* on board and is not a bad investment for any large yacht.

Tap. Tap the chest with the tip of a partially flexed finger. As with a tom-tom, the resonance of the chest is relative to the amount of air in the chest. Since the skin of the chest wall is not pulled tight like that on a snare drum, and since it is separated by several thicknesses of muscle and bone, this tone is normally of rather dull resonance, but not flat. Again, compare both sides. Use the uninjured side as a guide to the quality of the percussion note on the injured side. Are they the same? Is it hyperresonant (like a tom-tom) on one side or the other? Is it flat or dull on one side or the other? If you have ever watched a good marine surveyor "tap out" a hull, he is doing essentially the same thing. He uses a small hammer. You use your finger. As I describe various chest injuries, think in terms of what physical findings they might produce. Think in terms of our stoppered bottle as well, and always in terms of the ABCs of trauma: *airway, breathing, and circulation.*

HIGH-PRIORITY INJURIES

AIRWAY OBSTRUCTION

Clear and remove the obstruction.

PNEUMOTHORAX

A pneumothorax is a chest full of air. It is caused by a tear in the lung tissue that allows air to leak into the space between the lung and the chest wall. Remember our bottle? (See illustration 24.)

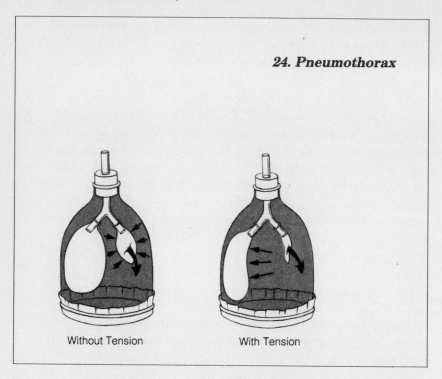

24. Pneumothorax

Without Tension   With Tension

This causes a collapse of the injured lung as the pleural space fills. The injury to the lung tissue can be caused by either blunt or penetrating trauma to the chest. It is also seen as a complication of scuba diving, where the lung "blows out" as one holds one's breath while ascending. (A no-no.) This allows the lung to overexpand as the pressure against it lessens. There are several types of pneumothoraces.

SIMPLE PNEUMOTHORAX

This generally involves a two-way leak, that is, air can ago in and out of the pleural space with respirations, or a very small leak. There may be shortness of breath and a "fluttery" feeling in the chest. On physical exam, breath sounds are *diminished or absent* on the involved side and the percussion noise is *hyperresonant.* The treatment of anything greater than a 10-percent pneumothorax requires a chest tube. If the victim is in no distress at rest, this can wait days for the proper medical help.

TENSION PNEUMOTHORAX

This type of pneumothorax is much more serious, may be lethal, and demands urgent treatment. It is essentially a one-way valve leak: Air is pulled into the pleural space with each breath and cannot exit when the victim breathes out. The lung becomes completely collapsed and pressure is exerted upon the heart and large blood vessels, as well as on the opposite lung, which is thus also endangered.

Tension pneumothorax is evidenced when the windpipe is shifted to the opposite side (to the right in illustration 24). There is also marked respiratory distress, absence of breath sounds on the involved side, distended neck veins, and a hyperresonant percussion note on the involved side. The victim will be blue (cyanotic) and gasping for breath. In this instance, emergency chest decompression is lifesaving.

Technique

Your medical kit should contain several *large-bore needles,* preferably 12 to 14 gauge. What must be done is to convert the tension pneumothorax into a simple pneumothorax by inserting this large-bore needle into the pleural space, allowing the air to escape. The needle should be inserted through skin prepared with antiseptic solutions and local anesthesia (such as lidocaine, Carbocaine), in the second or third spaces between two ribs in the mid-clavical line. This is one or two interspaces above the nipple in the line of the nipple. *Feel* the ribs, *feel* the space between them, and insert gery. If necessary, aspiration can be done using the same technique as described for pneumothorax but entering the chest lower, such as in the 8th interspace and aspirating gently the accumulated blood with a large syringe. The technique can be used repeatedly. This then is a lower-priority situation and, in the absence of respiratory distress, can be treated with rest, analgesics, and fluids until medical help can be found, that is, for several days.

FLAIL CHEST

As stated in the discussion of fractures, simple rib fractures are common, uncomfortable, generally uncomplicated, and heal spontaneously in "a matter of time." However, violent trauma to the chest wall can produce multiple rib fractures and destroy the bony integrity of the chest wall, interfering with the pressure gradients and mechanics of normal respiration, so that this "stoved-in" area of the chest wall moves independently. The motion is opposite that of normal breathing: The unstable section is pulled in on inspiration and moves out on expiration. (See illustrations 26 and 27.)

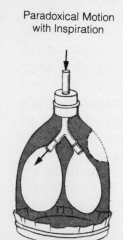
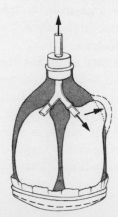

Paradoxical Motion
with Inspiration

26. *Flail Chest on Inspiration*
27. *Flail Chest on Expiration*

Breathing is decreased and oxygenation is diminished by this much less efficient bellows. The dynamics of circulation may also be altered by the pressure exerted on the midline structures in the chest, the heart and great vessels.

Emergency treatment involves splinting this flexible area with large gauze pads, sponge rubber, or any suitable material and firmly taping it in place with adhesive tape. This essentially fills in the caved-in portion of the chest wall and prevents paradoxical motion, although the result is a reduced space in that side of the chest. Medical help should be sought, analgesics given for pain. This injury alone, though dramatic and painful, can thus be effectively treated. However, it is rarely an isolated injury, and a hemothorax and/or pneumothorax may coincide with it, with their associated physical findings. (Remember them? Dullness to percussion with blood or fluid in the chest, hyperresonance with air; both will have diminished breath sounds.) Medical help should be sought on an urgent basis.

CHEST-WALL PAIN

On occasion, oral opiates or analgesics fail to alleviate chest-wall pain to the extent that coughing, which is essential for clearing mucus from the respiratory tract, is voluntarily suppressed because of the pain. Strapping can further reduce chest-wall movement, but intercostal nerve block may be necessary in these instances. The technique involves an injection of 2 to 3 cc of local anesthetic around the intercostal nerves, which run in a groove along the lower edge of each rib along with the intercostal blood vessels.

A small (22 to 25 gauge) needle, one or one and a half inches long, is inserted so as to make contact with the rib. (See illustration 28.)

The needle is advanced along the undersurface of the rib for a distance of .5 cm ($\frac{1}{4}''$) and should be perpendicular to the rib at this point.

CHAPTER 6

The Abdomen

The abdomen is like a stage
Enclosed within a fleshy cage.
The symptoms are the actors who,
Although they are a motley crew,
Act often with consummate art
The major or the minor part;
Nor do they usually say
Who is the author of the play.
That is for you to try and guess,
A problem which, I must confess,
Is made less easy from the fact
You seldom see the opening act,
And by the time that you arrive
The victim may be *just* alive.

The leading or principle symptoms are four;
They often are few, and seldom are more.
Though frequently minor ones come in and out
And make things more difficult, without a doubt
The "big" four I mean, whom you must watch well,
Most clearly the site of the author tell.
They come off the tongue in a simple refrain:
*Distention, rigidity, vomiting, pain.**

In no area of the body is the challenge of diagnosis as fascinating and demanding as with the abdomen. Fortunately, the important decisions are quite basic and revolve around the question "Does the patient need surgery or not, and if so, how soon?" In order to answer this basic question, a

The Diagnosis of the Acute Abdomen in Rhyme by Zeta, H. K. Lewis & Co. Ltd., London, 1955.

knowledge of the "big four" symptoms, how to elicit them, and what they signify, is essential.

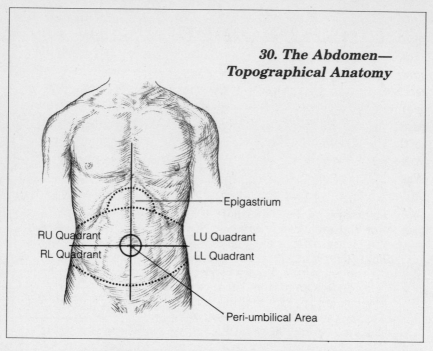

30. The Abdomen— Topographical Anatomy

Epigastrium

RU Quadrant

RL Quadrant

LU Quadrant

LL Quadrant

Peri-umbilical Area

PAIN

Since abdominal pain is most commonly the first complaint, it is important to evaluate its nature—its shape and form, so to speak. This is best done by *asking questions* about it. How and when did the pain start? Was it of a sudden or gradual onset? How long ago did it start? Did it follow any specific event such as eating or trauma? Is it related to motion or activity? Is it constant or intermittent? Is it crampy in nature, that is, does it build up to a peak and abate? Is it wavelike in occurrence? Is it sharp? Is it dull? Is there anything that makes it worse? Where is it? Does it radiate to any other spot? Is it localized to one spot? Is it generalized?

Answers to these questions give one a "pain profile" upon which further evaluations are based. The answers give hints to potential causes for the pain.

VOMITING

The act of vomiting is associated with many factors: *equilibrium* and balance (as in sea or motion sickness), *psychological factors* (as in repugnant sights or smells), *gastrointestinal irritation* (noxious agents, irritants, drugs), *cerebral factors* (increased intracranial pressure), *pain* (migraine, etc.), *obstruction* to the gastrointestinal tract. As with pain, the nature, timing, and quality of vomiting gives clues to the underlying disease process. The pattern is important. Was it associated with nausea? Was it voluminous or scant? Was it associated with pain? Did it *relieve pain*? Did it *relieve the nausea* if present? What were its physical characteristics—*color* (yellow, clear, dark, bloody?), *quality* (undigested food?) *timing* (just after eating?) Was it of rapid onset after pain? Was it preceded by long periods of nausea, or was the nausea sudden? Was it associated with diarrhea?

RIGIDITY

Rigidity is an involuntary tightness of the muscles of the abdominal wall. It makes the abdomen hard to the touch, resisting pressure or indentation of the abdominal wall by the examining hand. It is a reaction to *peritoneal irritation,* that is, irritation of the inner lining of the abdominal cavity (the peritoneum). It is a protective reaction as well. It may be generalized or localized, and its presence and location are significant. Generalized abdominal rigidity is seen with free peritonitis. Localized rigidity (spasm) is seen with localized peritonitis and is usually located over the inflamed organ or over an abscess.

ABDOMINAL DISTENTION

Protuberance or "bloating" of the abdomen is associated with ineffective propulsive action of the smooth muscle of the intestines. Its significance in intestinal obstruction will be discussed later. The abdomen becomes protuberant and enlarged in girth. Again, question the patient about associated pain and vomiting. Is the pain crampy or constant? Is the distention associated with flatulence or diarrhea? Distended bowl is *tender* to palpation. Otherwise the intestine itself is insensitive to pain. Distention may be *mechanical,* as when obstruction is present, or *paralytic,* where propulsive action of the bowel is absent because of a chemical or neurological imbalance. Mechanical obstruction demands intervention. Paralytic ileus does not. As you can see, the distinction is not always easy—especially without X rays.

ABDOMINAL TRAUMA

Injuries to the abdomen generally fall into two categories: *blunt,* due to a blow or concussive force to the abdomen, and *penetrating,* due to sharp, piercing wounds to the abdomen.

BLUNT TRAUMA

A blow to the abdomen usually involves a fall from a height or direct concussion, for example, by a fist or a freely swinging mast. Other injuries are frequently associated, and a careful history and examination of the injury are essential. The dynamics involve the compression of intra-abdominal organs against solid vertebrae, which can cause rupture both of hollow, air-containing organs and of solid organs such as liver, spleen, kidney, and—rarely—pancreas. Hollow organs (stomach, intestine) leak intestinal contents into the abdominal (peritoneal) cavity, such as bile or gastric juice, which is highly acid and irritating. Rupture of the colon (large intestine) causes bacteria-laden fecal material to infect the abdominal cavity, causing peritonitis and death if untreated.

Solid organs bleed, and blood in the abdominal cavity is an irritant as well, causing peritonitis. The blood loss itself can cause shock, its severity depending on how fast the blood is lost.

The abdominal wall is swathed in muscles. These muscles are protective, so injury to the abdominal wall can cause muscular rigidity and pain. These effects must be differentiated from the pain of internal bleeding, infections, or chemical irritation to the peritoneum—which is the inner lining of the abdominal cavity and is sensitive to pain.

Abdominal-wall pain can easily be distinguished from intra-abdominal pain. If the victim is asked to tense the muscles of his abdomen by lifting his legs up together or by lifting his head and shoulders up (as with a partial "sit-up"), the tenderness to palpation of the abdomen when there is injury to the abdominal wall is usually *equal* whether the muscles are tight or relaxed. Injury within the peritoneal cavity usually elicits *more tenderness when the muscles are relaxed.*

Evaluation of a person who has sustained blunt abdominal injury involves, as with the chest, the use of our senses. *Look* for bruising and abrasions. *Listen* to see if the normal "gurgling" of the intestines, well known to all of us (especially at mealtimes), is present. These sounds disappear with peritonitis from any cause. *Feel* for tenderness. Tenderness may be *direct,* that is, in response to direct pressure of the examining fingers over a specific area, or it may be *referred,* that is, palpation in the lower left abdomen may elicit pain in the lower right abdomen. Since it's all "pain" to the examinee, one must ask, "Where do you feel the pain when I press here?"

Pain may also be *indirect* or "rebound": Sudden release of pressure by the examining finger may elicit sharp pain. This is a reliable sign of peritoneal irritation and is helpful in differentiating peritonitis from other painful abdominal conditions. Pain on *coughing* is of similar significance, and is basically an indirect method of eliciting rebound tenderness. Blunt abdominal trauma can also cause *shearing* forces, which can tear blood vessels and cause intra-abdominal hemorrhage.

SPLENIC INJURY

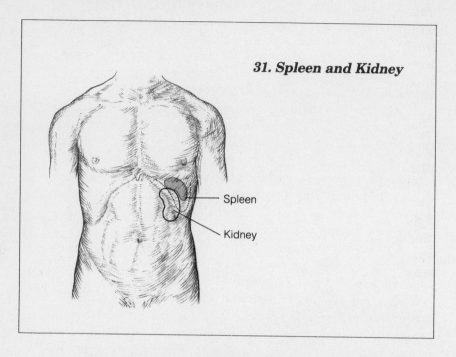

31. Spleen and Kidney

Spleen

Kidney

The organ in the abdomen most frequently injured by blunt trauma is the spleen, which is located in the left upper quadrant of the abdomen, tucked under the ribs just above the left kidney. Fractures of the overlying ribs are frequently associated with splenic injuries. The spleen may be "bruised," with collection of blood under its capsule, or it may be *frankly ruptured,* and can cause massive hemorrhage and death if untreated. Until recently, surgeons removed spleens with abandon. However, the spleen has been shown to have important functions in fighting infection, and surgeons today try to preserve the spleen when possible, and to repair it if surgery is necessary to stop bleeding.

Another important fact to remember is that the spleen, when bruised, can rupture and bleed days or weeks later (so called "delayed rupture" of the spleen). The threat of serious hemorrhage exists, then, for weeks after a splenic injury.

Diagnosis is often difficult. Classically, a history of blunt trauma to the left upper quadrant of the abdomen, or a blow across the lower ribs of the back such as might occur with a swinging boom, associated with left-upper-quadrant pain, tenderness to deep palpation, muscular rigidity, *"referred"* pain to the left shoulder (Kehr's sign) and evidence of bleeding (rapid heart rate, lowered blood pressure, and pallor) all indicate splenic injury with bleeding. Other injuries can confuse the picture (fractured ribs with pain on respiration or touch), unconsciousness from a head injury, as well as injuries to other intra-abdominal organs).

This is a high-priority injury. If the person is not "shocky," he should be made to rest and medical help sought. If the person shows signs of shock, *intravenous* fluids (saline Ringer's lactate) should be started—until facilities for blood transfusion can be attained. The only way to control splenic hemorrhage is *surgically*.

LIVER INJURY

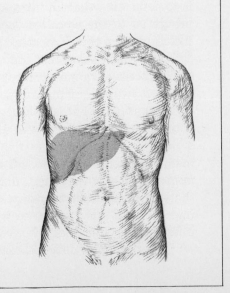

32. Liver

may seem obvious that probing of these wounds might give some information as to the wound depth. Don't be misled. A probe has been described as a long thin instrument with a blunted tip on one end and an idiot on the other. Never use a probe in this situation. Most information can be gained from gently examining the wound with a sterile, gloved hand and finger, even if the skin has to be anesthetized with local anesthesia to do this. It should best be done by a physician or surgeon.

ACUTE INFLAMMATION

APPENDICITIS

This is the most common inflammatory condition to involve the abdomen and, since common things occur commonly, one that should be thought of initially in someone complaining of abdominal pain with no history of trauma.

Appendicitis can mimic many other diseases. However, the "typical" case usually complains of pain about the area of the navel, which gradually migrates to the right lower quadrant of the abdomen, where it stays. The patient may have nausea and vomiting, and less commonly, diarrhea. He is usually not hungry, and the pain, though constant, is made worse by walking or coughing. The pain is localized to an area between the iliac crest and the navel (see illustration 33).

On examination, tenderness is most marked in this area, and pressure on other areas may be perceived as painful in the right lower quadrant (direct referred tenderness). Similarly, rebound tenderness may be direct, as well as referred from other areas—McBurney's point. Muscle spasm and involuntary guarding of the area are present to some degree.

Fever, if present, is usually not greater than 101° F in the uncomplicated "typical" case. All types of variations on this theme can occur in this disease—and the diagnosis can, at times, be extremely difficult. The disease is usually more acute and rapidly progressive in the young and the elderly.

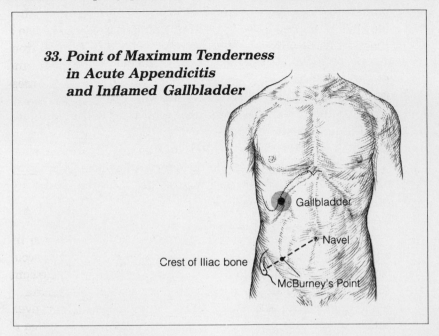

33. Point of Maximum Tenderness in Acute Appendicitis and Inflamed Gallbladder

Gallbladder

Navel

Crest of Iliac bone

McBurney's Point

THE GALLBLADDER

The gallbladder, which is a storage sac for bile, resides in the right upper quadrant of the abdomen, where it is in intimate contact with the liver. It pokes out just below the margin of the rib cage on the right. It has a muscular wall that, when stimulated *by eating,* contracts and "squirts" bile into the intestine to help in the digestion of food, especially fats. Stones (calculi) in the gallbladder are usually formed from bile salts or cholesterol and irritate the sac that contains them, causing an inflammatory response (cholecystitis) and acute symptoms. Classically, an "attack" occurs after ingestion of a fatty meal and consists of pain, sometimes wavelike or colicky in nature, limited generally to the right upper quadrant of the abdomen. Vomiting is a frequent associated sign. Shoulder pain is also seen, and is referred pain, thought to be due to irritation of the diaphragm. Fever may develop.

In many instances, a gallbladder attack will subside spontaneously in twenty-four to forty-eight hours. If symptoms progress, however, and become more severe, with persistent pain, vomiting, and fever, medical help should be sought. Demerol will often completely relieve the pain. Don't use morphine. It can make the attack worse by causing spasm of the ductal system that promotes emptying of the gallbladder. If there is an inordinate delay, broad-spectrum antibiotics such as tetracycline, which are effective against a wide variety of organisms, should be started. Efforts should be made to prevent dehydration with clear, nonfatty liquids by mouth.

GASTROENTERITIS

Appendicitis and gallbladder disease are frequent "surgical" conditions that affect younger age groups. However, gastroenteritis, which should not have surgical implications, is the most frequent inflammatory condition in any environment. It is characterized by its nonspecificity—diffuse, crampy abdominal pain, which is generally nonlocalizing—and its association with vomiting and diarrhea. Fever is absent or low grade. Gastroenteritis responds to food restriction—fluids (preferably clear) only, by mouth—and to a variety of intestinal antispasmodic medications (belladonna, Donnatal, Bentyl). This illness can be viral or bacterial. It can be severe if associated with spoiled food (salmonellosis), and dehydration can occur rapidly in severe cases. Intravenous fluids may be necessary, as well as antibiotics, if the illness does not respond to conservative measures.

MAL DE MER (MOTION SICKNESS, SEASICKNESS)

The nemesis of all seamen, seasickness is poorly understood. A multiplicity of factors are involved in this "motion sickness." There is little question that the balance (vestibular) mechanisms of the inner ear are involved. Psychological factors such as fear and anxiety also play an important role: It is not unusual for seasoned yachtsmen to become seasick during storms, when anxiety and tension are high. However, I have seen people "turn green" when coming aboard a stable yacht tied to a floating dock. It is therefore difficult to make generalized statements regarding the exact cause of the illness. Certain generalities can be made about therapy, however. The new systems for absorbing scopolamine through the skin seem to be quite effective and avoid the obvious difficulty of "getting pills down" when nauseated or vomiting as well as the inconvenience of using suppositories. Transderm-Scōp can be used as a preventive measure in the seasick-prone sailor and side effects seem to be minimal. Simply stick the patch to the skin and the medicine is absorbed. There is less drowsiness than with Dramamine. Some visual reference to the horizon often helps as does the fresh air topside. The worst place for someone is "below" in heaving seas. Dry crackers (Saltines or plain dry biscuits) seem to help the nausea.

CHAPTER 7

Eye Injuries

The eye is, in general, a well-protected organ. It sits in a bony cup (the orbit), on a cushion of fat. Its exposed surface is protected by eyelids and lashes and is covered by a durable transparent membrane (the cornea). This membrane has the ability to regenerate rapidly and usually heals without scarring unless its deeper layers are injured. The eye is also protected by a highly sensitive nerve supply, and it has its own built-in irrigation system (tears). The eye is also relatively easy to examine.

In spite of these built-in protective mechanisms, the eye is frequently injured. These injuries can be roughly classified as nonpenetrating or penetrating.

NONPENETRATING INJURIES

ABRASION

This is actually a scratch on the cornea, eyelid, or conjunctiva (the outer surface of the cornea that extends to the insides of upper and lower lids). These injuries rarely require surgical treatment but may produce severe pain associated with profuse tearing, blinking, redness, and sometimes inability to open the eye, in which case a drop of local anesthetic such as 0.5% tetracaine may facilitate examination. This drug should not be used repeatedly because it delays normal healing. Any debris should be removed, either by irrigation or mechanically with a cotton swab. Antibiotic drops or ointment (Chloromycetin Ophthalmic, 1%) will prevent potential bacterial infection. An eye patch, applied with firm but gentle pressure, will make the eye comfortable and should be left on for one to three days, with daily changes and use of the antibiotic.

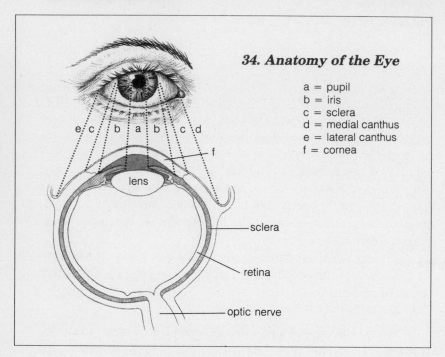

34. Anatomy of the Eye

a = pupil
b = iris
c = sclera
d = medial canthus
e = lateral canthus
f = cornea

FOREIGN BODIES

These are a frequent cause of eye injury. Windborne objects, chips or flakes of metal, wood, or glass, are the most frequent offenders. Those containing iron may cause a ring of rust that penetrates the cornea. These objects cause pain, watery eyes, and a sensation that "something is in one's eye." The eye reddens and frequent blinking occurs. Again, a local anesthetic may be needed to see it. If the foreign body is loose, it can usually be picked up by a sterile cotton swab or Q-Tip. A sterile hypodermic needle may gently lift it out. Deeper foreign bodies may have to be removed surgically.

Following their removal, antibiotic ointment applied three times a day may be necessary for several days. An eye patch may or may not be needed. Examining the undersurface of the lids is best done by depressing the lower lid, or by everting the upper lid by using an applicator and folding the lid back on itself.

CONTUSIONS

A blunt blow to the eye can result in hemorrhage in the eyelids ("black eye") or under the conjunctiva, edema (swelling) or even rupture of the cornea, or hemorrhage into the anterior chamber of the eye. Severe blunt trauma can lead to rupture of the eyeball itself. Any injury that involves bleeding into the eye may cause permanent damage. Such an injury requires absolute bed rest for four to five days with both eyes bandaged and the bed elevated 60 degrees to prevent further hemorrhage. Black eyes normally require no special treatment. If there is a reduction in vision, suspect a more severe injury and seek proper medical help.

BURNS

Burns are most commonly due to ultraviolet radiation, infrared radiation, heat (thermal injury), or chemicals. In sailing, **ultraviolet radiation** from exposure to the sun is the most common burn. Pain and inability to tolerate light (photophobia) usually come after a latent period of several hours after exposure. A "haziness" in vision may be experienced. Treatment includes antibiotics and an eye patch. Cold compresses may help for comfort.

Thermal burns usually affect the eyelids and cause swelling and pain. Antibiotics and dressings are indicated.

Chemical burns should be treated immediately. Alkali burns are more serious than acid burns since they penetrate the cornea. Irrigate with lots of fresh water immediately—if available. If not, over the side and into the drink, the sooner the better. After irrigation, antibiotics, analgesics by mouth, if necessary, and eye patches should be used. Consult an ophthalmologist if possible.

PENETRATING INJURIES

All penetrating injuries (lacerations, perforations, penetrating foreign bodies) require good medical help. *Do not* use antibiotic ointment while awaiting help. Antibiotic *drops* are okay. Both eyes should be patched, since movement of the good eye may harm the injured eye. (Our eyes move together.) Surgical repair will be necessary and the prognosis will depend on the extent of the injury and the quality of the surgeon.

INJURIES NEAR THE EYE

THE EYELID

If the edge of the lid is lacerated, suture correction must be accurately done to prevent notching of the eyelids. This is not a threatening emergency unless there are associated injuries, whether to the globe itself or to the person. However, medical help should be sought for primary repair. These wounds should not be left open. They should be thoroughly evaluated by an opthalmologist for related injuries, which may be more extensive than is apparent on first inspection.

FRACTURE OF THE ORBITAL RIM

This is significant if the muscles attached to the eye, which control coordinated eye movements, become trapped in fractures of the orbital rim. This produces a restriction in the mobility of the eye, and necessitates surgical repair. Although this is not a prime emergency and can wait several days, steps should be taken to obtain medical advice. Special

X rays are usually needed. Ignored, these fractures can lead to permanent injury. Double vision or inability to move the eye in a complete free range are clues to the existence of such a fracture.

INFECTIONS

THE EYELIDS

Infections involving the tear duct or **tear sac of the lower lid** (dacryocystitis) usually involve obstruction of the tear duct, which is located at the inner corner of each eye. Pain, swelling, redness, and tenderness are localized to the skin over the sac. Pussy material may be expressed from the duct or sac. Treatment includes systemic antibiotics: penicillin (1 to 2 million units per day intramuscularly) or ampicillin (2 gm daily orally or intramuscularly) or tetracycline (1 gm daily orally for seven days. *Warm saline soaks,* in the form of compresses, help to cleanse the area and reduce redness and swelling.

Infections of the lids (**sty, hordeolum**) usually involve the glands in the lids. Treat with a local antibiotic and warm compresses.

Infections of the **orbit** may follow an acute sinus infection. These can be very serious. The eye becomes swollen, protuberant, and tender. Motion of the eye is difficult and painful. Therapy involves administration of large doses of antibiotics intramuscularly or intravenously (20 million units of penicillin per day or cephalothin, 4.0 gm per day in divided doses). If fever, chills, headache, nausea, vomiting, and sleepiness occur, suspect a "cavernous sinus thrombosis," usually secondary to a bloodborne infection from the throat, nose, or face (don't squeeze pimples on the face). Again, aggressive therapy with massive doses of antibiotics is indicated.

CONJUNCTIVITIS

This common affliction of the eye—known as pinkeye—has multiple causes, viral, bacterial, fungal, parasitic, or allergic. Signs of conjunctival infection are discharge, tearing, redness, and itching. *Itching* is most severe in allergic conjunctivitis. *Discharge* is most severe in bacterial conjunctivitis. *Tearing* is most severe in viral conjunctivitis. *Redness* is universal to all.

All are generally treated locally with antibiotics or antifungal agents (Mycostatin). Local steroids as well as antibiotics help in allergic conjunctivitis. Mild decongestant eyedrops (Vasocon, Albalon) may relieve acute symptoms.

CHAPTER 8

Urologic and OB/GYN Emergencies

An axiom of medicine is "Never say never and never say always." What this means is that there are *always* exceptions to the rules, and there are *never* absolutes when dealing with the human animal.

Almost everything in this book so far has been unisex. Now we must discuss some emergencies that are peculiar to one or the other sex. These include prostatitis in the male, and cystitis, which is much more frequent in the female although not unheard of in males. (Symptoms are similar, as is treatment.) I will also cover kidney stones, other urinary-tract infections, renal trauma, and some gynecologic problems.

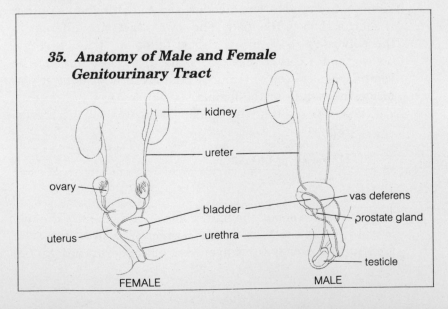

35. Anatomy of Male and Female Genitourinary Tract

kidney

ureter

ovary

vas deferens

prostate gland

bladder

uterus

urethra

testicle

FEMALE   MALE

Basic Anatomy

The urogenital tract in the male normally consists of paired kidneys, each with its own drainage system, the ureters, which empty into the bladder, which acts as a reservoir for urine as well as a muscular sac to expel urine. From the bladder in the male, the single exit pathway is the urethra, which runs through the prostate gland at the base of the bladder and out through the penis.

The kidneys are well protected in the flanks, under the ribs, the liver on the right and the spleen on the left. Strong muscles of the back also protect them. The bladder is protected by its position in the "hollow" of the pelvis. It becomes more exposed, of course, when it is distended and rises out of the pelvis—at least its uppermost portion (dome). The prostate lies just below the bladder, behind the pubic bone. This structure is composed of many glands, which drain into the urethra as it passes through the prostate. In the same region, the vas deferens, the tube that carries sperm from the testicles, enters into the urethra. Sperm and prostatic secretions make up the ejaculate.

In the female, the upper tracts are similar, that is, two kidneys, two ureters, one bladder, and an exiting urethra that is shorter than in the male. The lower tracts are different in the pelvis. Paired ovaries, paired fallopian tubes, a single uterus, and a cervix that forms the uppermost limit of the vagina complete the differences. The urethral opening is just inside the vagina in the female.

One can see that the bladder is in front of the uterus.

KIDNEY STONES

Stones are one of the most common afflictions of the urinary tract and can form in any portion of it, from kidney to urethra, and/or they can travel from above downward. Stones

may be small and pass spontaneously, or they may be large
and cause obstructions and kidney damage. Stones tend to re-
cur, so a history of previous stones may be available. *If* stones
are passed, they should be saved for analysis if possible, since
information on their chemical makeup may help to prevent
recurrence by suggesting alterations in diet. This may entail
changing the pH (acidity/alkalinity) of the urine and/or the
intake of foods that may cause increased urinary excretion of
certain chemical compounds. Kidney stones may also give a
clue to underlying diseases. Symptoms depend on where the
stone lodges.

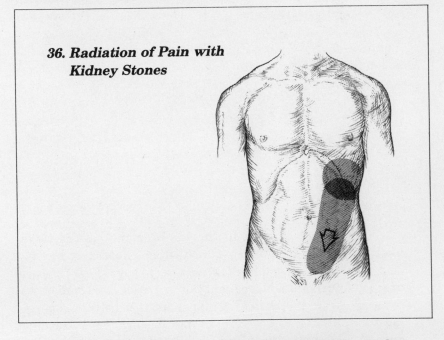

**36. Radiation of Pain with
Kidney Stones**

A stone located **between kidney and bladder** is the
most symptomatic. It produces *dull flank pain* and *colic* (due
to smooth muscle spasm), as well as nausea, vomiting, abdominal distention, and mechanical ileus (see p. 86). If infection intervenes above the obstructed area, fever and chills
occur. The pain of renal (kidney-related) colic can be totally
disabling. It radiates from flank to groin. (See illustration 36.)

In women it may radiate to the vulvar area. In men, the pain may be felt in the bladder, scrotum, or testicle. This is because the same nerves supply both the upper ureter and testicle. On the right side the pain may mimic appendicitis. Pain is usually sudden in onset, and the agonizing, colicky, radiating pain may be accompanied by a dull constant ache in the flank and in the angle where the ribs meet the backbone (the costovertebral angle). (See illustration 37.)

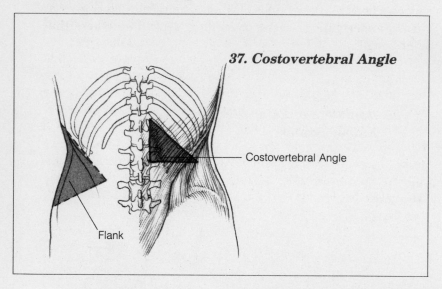

37. Costovertebral Angle

Costovertebral Angle

Flank

If the stone is close to the **bladder** the pain is more likely to radiate to the scrotum or vulva. Blood may be evident in the urine; small clots may be passed. Symptoms of urgency to urinate and frequency of urination are common as the stone nears the bladder. The patient is usually in agonizing pain, unable to get comfortable (pacing, etc.). He may have cold, clammy skin. There is marked tenderness over the costovertebral angle area and the flank. Fever may be present and indicates infection.

Treatment

Eighty percent of stones in the ureter will pass spontaneously. Treat with analgesics (morphine, Demerol), antispasmodics (atropine, Banthine), and large amounts of fluid by mouth. Physical activity should be encouraged. Hot packs to the area of pain sometimes help. If these do not bring relief, seek medical help. Fever indicating infection indicates the use of urinary antibiotics such as Gantrisin.

BLADDER STONES

These are commonly caused by infection, but they may occur spontaneously. There may be more than one. Since it takes time for stones to develop, the symptoms may be chronic. However, the male patient may complain of sudden cessation of the urinary stream, associated with pain radiating down the penis, as the stone blocks the outflow of the bladder. Bloody or cloudy urine may ensue. The cloudiness is due to infection. Complete urinary obstruction may be caused by a stone lodging in the urethra, but smaller stones may pass. General treatment includes analgesics for pain and antibiotics to control infection until the stone(s) can be removed. The presence of urinary obstruction indicates an emergency condition.

URINARY TRACT INJURIES

Generally, injuries to the kidney and bladder are related to blunt abdominal trauma (85 percent), and they are hardly ever isolated injuries. Associated abdominal-organ injuries are present in 80 percent of renal wounds. Falls and fights, guns and knives, are the most common causes, other than rapid deceleration injuries—not likely to occur on shipboard unless one is decelerating on the deck from a rapid trip down the mast. Falls in a pitchy sea against stanchions or winches may produce direct blows to the kidney or bladder. Falling from a height and landing on one's buttocks has been known to produce indirect renal injury.

Fortunately, the kidneys are surrounded by a strong fibrous envelope that has the ability to confine most hematomas that may surround the kidney. However, the blood vessels to the kidneys are subjected to trauma from torsion and tearing. (Blood in the urine is generally the first sign of renal injury.)

Bladder injuries are usually associated with pelvic fractures, blunt and violent trauma. Shock, necessitating resuscitation, is the rule, rather than the exception. Those so injured are critically ill and need prompt medical attention. Bloody urine is the first sign of kidney or bladder injury, especially bladder injury. There may be small amounts of blood in the urine with extensive injury, and vice versa, so that diagnosis does not depend on quantity.

Blood in the urine following renal trauma demands investigation; following bladder injury it demands *immediate* investigation. These injuries should be treated professionally.

URINARY INFECTIONS

CYSTITIS

This is far more common in women than in men, and the bladder infection is caused by bacteria entering the bladder from the urethra. Symptoms usually occur one and a half to two days after intercourse and manifest themselves by difficulty in urinating, with burning, urgency (incontinence), frequency of urination, and frequent nighttime urination. Sometimes a little blood may be noticed on the toilet tissue. Fever is usually absent.

In men cystitis can be the result of a quiescent prostate infection. It may follow sexual excitement or alcoholic overindulgence. Symptoms are the same—and in men, prostatitis may cause identical symptoms, although a preceding urethral discharge may imply prostatitis or venereal disease.

Treatment

Specific measures involve antibiotics (Nitrofurantoin, ampicillin, penicillin G, tetracycline or sulfonamides (such as Gantrisin). Plenty of fruit juices, which alkalize the urine, or sodium bicarbonate (16 to 20 gm) may help relieve the irritable bladder. Warm sitz baths also relieve the discomfort. In women who suffer recurrent attacks of cystitis following intercourse, postcoital voiding with force will help to abolish the infection.

PROSTATITIS

This is usually caused by bacterial infection. Symptoms are similar to those of cystitis: burning on urination, frequent urination (day and night), aching low-back pain, or lower abdominal pain. Fever and cloudy urine are common. Blood may appear at the end of urination. If the prostate gland becomes markedly swollen, urinary retention (inability to urinate) may occur.

Treatment

Antibiotics, namely erythromycin, Cefazolin, cephalexin, or a combination of sulfamethoxazole, 16 mg, and trimethoprim, 800 mg, work effectively, and a response should be seen within a few days. The pain may require analgesics such as Tylenol or Percocet. Warm sitz baths can be comforting. Avoid all the things you like—sex, alcohol, and spicy foods—until the symptoms subside.

URETHRITIS

This is an infection of the male urethra, usually bacterial and marked by a discharge from the penis—which should be perfectly obvious to the person who has it. It may be very profuse in gonorrheal urethritis.

Treatment

Antibiotics, such as sulfonamide combined with erythromycin or tetracycline, are effective. Avoid intercourse, since it prolongs the acute phase of the disease.

DOSAGE SCHEDULES

Sulfonamides (Sulfisoxazole, Trisulfapyramine) are drugs of choice for acute urinary infections. Dose is 2 to 4 *grams* per day (15 mg per kgm of weight for children) given in divided doses for 7 to 10 days orally.

Trimethoprim: 100 mg by mouth every 8 to 12 hours

Trimethoprim-Sulfamethoxazole (co-trimoxazole) fixed combination (400 mg sulfa and 80 mg trimethoprim): 2 tablets three times a day

Pencillins: Penicillin G: 800,000 units 4 times a day
Ampicillin 500 mg 4 times a day

Cephalosporins: 250 mg to 1 gm every 6 hours

Tetracycline: 0.5 gm 4 times a day—high resistance rate. Not for general urinary tract use, but *good* for gonorrhea (5-day therapy). Absorption impaired by milk, antacids, iron. *Not for use in pregnant women or children under 7.*

Spectinomycin: (intramuscular only) single dose of 2 gm cures 95% of gonorrheal infections. PAINFUL SHOT!!

Erythromycin (like penicillin—*useable* in penicillin-allergic patient): 300 mg orally 3 to 4 times a day

Urinary antiseptics: Drugs that concentrate mainly in the genitourinary tract with little general body effects. **Nitrofurantoin:** 100 mg 4 times daily by mouth

KIDNEY INFECTIONS

These serious infections are usually due to bacterial infections ascending to the kidney from the bladder. A history of repeated infections is common. The onset of symptoms is rapid, over several hours, and consists of pain over the flank(s), aching in character and severe in intensity. Pain may radiate to the lower abdomen. Symptoms of cystitis may precede or follow the kidney pain. Nausea, vomiting, and diarrhea may occur. Fever and chills are common (101° F, 38° C). Rapid heart rate may occur. Tenderness usually is present over the involved kidney. Bowel sounds may be diminished. These people look and feel quite sick. Treatment should be based on urine cultures. If these are unobtainable, an empirical choice of a safe, effective drug such as ampicillin or tetracycline should be started. Pain should be relieved by appropriate drugs (Percocet, Darvon, Demerol) and an antispasmodic, (belladonna, Donnatal). Bed rest and adequate fluid intake should lead to a decline in symptoms in forty-eight to seventy-two hours. If not, medical help should be sought and the antibiotics should be changed. Kidney X rays should be taken *at a medical facility.*

GYNECOLOGIC EMERGENCIES

Injuries to the normal, nonpregnant female pelvic organs are exceedingly rare. The uterus, fallopian tubes, and ovaries are well protected in the pelvis from most trauma. Blunt trauma is almost unheard of, and penetrating injuries are unusual. Gunshot wounds are the most common injuries. Pelvic fractures or lacerations of the vagina and/or urethra from straddle-type accidents, sexual activity, or foreign bodies are other common injuries to the female genitalia.

In the pregnant female, one of the major threats is from blunt abdominal trauma. Being thrown against a stationary object—countertop, stanchion, pedestal, or bulkhead—in a heavy sea may pose a risk to the very pregnant female (very pregnant = third trimester). Although the pregnant uterus is a bigger target, it is also protective to organs behind it, and it is fluid filled and therefore shock absorbing. Injury to the fetus is caused by objects penetrating the uterus. These are usually fatal to both mother and fetus.

SPONTANEOUS ABORTIONS

Abortions are mentioned here because there may be similarities to ectopic pregnancy and understanding abortion may give more insight into the diagnosis of one or the other.

Abortion is the expulsion of the products of conception before the fetus is mature enough to live ("miscarriage"). The causes of abortions are multiple and beyond the scope of this manual. The condition is suspected when any woman who might be pregnant experiences irregularities in uterine bleeding. This is usually followed by increased bleeding, eventually cramplike pain, and the expulsion of tissue from the uterus.

Spontaneous abortion occurs naturally and may be complete—all the products of conception are expelled—or incomplete—only a portion of these products are expelled and bleeding continues. In either case, medical help should be sought, although a spontaneous complete abortion is not necessarily an extreme emergency. The woman should be urged to rest. Tampons should be avoided and sexual relations should be avoided, both for at least one week. Some bleeding may occur spottily for ten to fourteen days. Raised temperature, excessive bleeding (heavier than the heaviest period), chills, or prolonged abdominal pain demand urgent medical advice. In extreme cases, hemorrhage may cause shock, and supportive therapy should be started by placing the patient in the head-down, feet-elevated position, conserving body heat with blankets, and administering Ringer's solution intravenously. Oxygen, if available, should be administered. It is crucial for the patient in shock to be treated *promptly*.

CHAPTER 9

Medical Seamanship

BASIC LIFE SUPPORT

Basic life support is an emergency first-aid procedure involving the recognition of airway obstruction, respiratory arrest, or cardiac arrest, followed by the proper application of cardiopulmonary resuscitation (CPR). CPR involves establishing and maintaining an open airway, providing artificial respiration (by mouth to mouth or mouth to airway), and providing artificial circulation by means of external compression of the heart.

Advanced life support is basic life support plus the use of auxiliary equipment and techniques such as insertion of a breathing tube into the windpipe, intravenous fluids, drugs, cardiac monitors, respirators, etc.

Some of the techniques normally referred to as advanced life support have been mentioned in this book, but the teaching of these techniques is beyond our scope. Some skippers may have already mastered some of these techniques and therefore reference to them is included. Those not so well trained should view the references to such techniques as a definite indication to seek more sophisticated medical help. Admittedly, knowing what is needed and not being able to do it is a terrible frustration. However, anyone who is putting to sea for a prolonged time, isolated from the mainstream of the world and modern medical facilities, must evaluate his preparedness to take on responsibility for the sick or injured who may accompany him.

As impressive as the modern ambulance is, basic life support is straightforward and uncomplicated and requires no burdensome or sophisticated equipment. Because of the urgency of the situations in which these skills may be needed, familiarity with the techniques described in this chapter should be learned beforehand. The oxygen needs of the brain will not wait for the reader to pursue this chapter leisurely. Practice beforehand makes things a lot easier, and may save a life.

RECOGNIZING THE PROBLEM

(Follow these directions as illustrated in the Life Support Decision Tree on page 118.)

In cases of a collapsed or unconscious person, the decision to start CPR is based on two yes or no questions:

Is the person breathing?
Is there a pulse?

To answer these questions rapidly and to immediately start CPR is paramount—and involves using your senses.

Look for motion of the chest.
Listen for air exiting from the nose or mouth.
Feel for the carotid pulse in the neck, just below and deep to the angle of the jawbone.

If respirations are present, simply maintain an open airway. If not, open the airway. This is done by first tilting the person's head backward as far as possible (head tilt) with the person lying on his back. The rescuer places one hand beneath the victim's neck and the other hand on his forehead and tilts the head backward. (See illustration 38.)

This maneuver extends the neck and lifts the tongue away from the back of the throat. This method is effective in most cases. In some cases, adding forward displacement of the lower jaw may be also necessary (jaw thrust). Always make certain that there is nothing in the mouth: Sweep your finger around inside the mouth to make certain there are no foreign bodies.

38. Head Tilt Maneuver

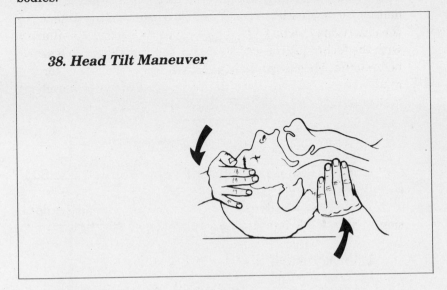

If the victim is now breathing spontaneously you (and the victim) are in good shape. If no respirations are occurring, then mouth-to-mouth rescue breathing must be started—NOW!! Maintain the head tilt, close the nose with a pinch between thumb and forefinger, cover the victim's mouth with your own, and give four deep breaths. LOOK to see if the chest moves during this inflation of the lungs. If so, continue rescue breathing. If the chest does *not* move, reevaluate the airway. Give a sharp blow to the middle of the upper back, make sure the throat is clear, and attempt rescue breathing again—until the chest moves.

Regarding the pulse: If there is a pulse present, continue breathing for the victim or maintaining his airway if breathing is present. If no pulse is present, a sharp blow to the chest may start cardiac action. The blow is with the smooth side of the fist, delivered to the middle of the breastbone from eight to twelve inches above the chest. (See illustration 39.)

If this fails to start the heart, then external cardiac compression must be started.

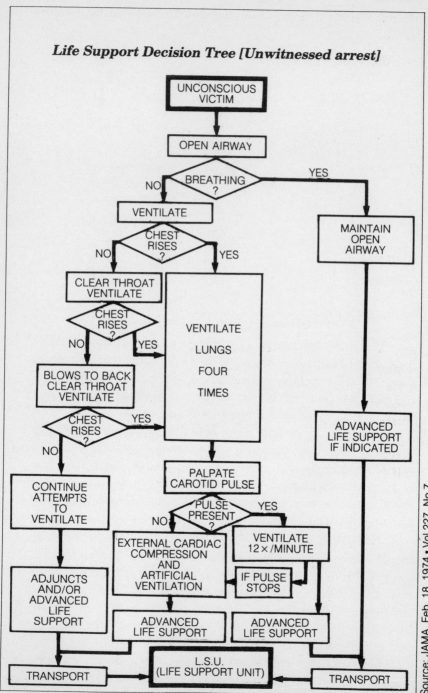

Life Support Decision Tree [Unwitnessed arrest]

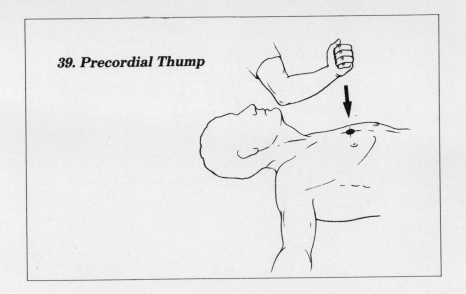

39. Precordial Thump

EXTERNAL CARDIAC COMPRESSION

Artificial respiration is *always* required when external cardiac compression (ECC) is used. The victim must be horizontal and leg elevation, if this is possible, may help carry blood to the brain. The position of the rescuer(s) is depicted in illustrations 40–41.

Kneeling close to the victim's side, he places the long axis of the heel of one hand over the long axis of the lower half of the breastbone (practice! practice! practice!) one to one and a half inches *above* the end of the breastbone (toward the victim's head). The other hand is placed over the first one, and the rescuer then leans forward over the victim so that his arms are piston-straight and vertical pressure is exerted from the shoulders down to depress the breastbone a minimum of one and a half to two inches. Remember to compress and then relax completely so that the breastbone comes back to its normal position. Relaxation follows compression in a rhythmic, smooth tempo—the rate of which is determined by the number of rescuers. (See illustrations 40 and 41.)

For two rescuers the compression rate is 60 per minute.

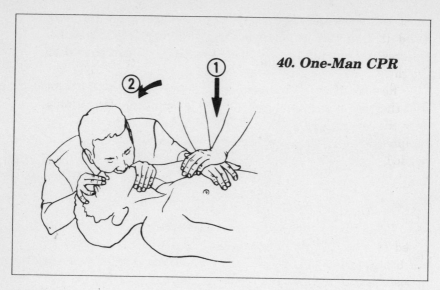

40. One-Man CPR

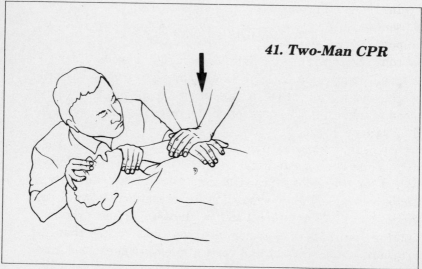

41. Two-Man CPR

One breath should be given for each 5 compressions without interruption of compression. Timing is important—and verbal counting helps.

One rescuer must perform both ECC and breathing at a rate of two quick lung breaths after each 15 chest compressions. The chest compressions must be more rapid (80/minute) to compensate for giving fewer breaths. One rescuer can become exhausted rapidly, so help should be sought.

Resuscitation of infants and children is similar except that the heel of one hand only is used for children. For infants only the tips of the index and middle fingers are needed for compression and only three quarters of an inch depression is needed.

EVALUATING CPR

The ability of the pupils of the eye to constrict when exposed to bright light indicates adequate oxygen delivery to the brain. Pupils that are widely dilated and remain so when exposed to light indicate poor or no oxygenation to the brain—and either death or inadequate CPR. The continued presence of fixed, dilated pupils after prolonged CPR with no response obviously indicates failure. In general, CPR should be continued until:

- Effective circulation and respiration is restored, or
- A physician or properly trained medical personnel (EMTs, paramedics) assume the care of the victim, or
- The rescuer becomes exhausted and is unable to continue.

If possible, the decision to discontinue CPR should be a medical one.

DROWNING

Basic life-support resuscitation following drowning is essentially the same as described for cardiac or respiratory failure except for certain special considerations. Ideally one would like to start resuscitation as soon as the drowning victim is reached. It is impossible to start ECC in the water, however, and mouth-to-mouth or mouth-to-nose resuscitation is extremely difficult unless one can float the victim's head on some object. Artificial respiration should be started as soon as the rescuer can stand (or kneel). Also, drowning victims swallow and/or breathe in large quantities of water—which impairs adequate respiration. Turn the victim over, belly down, and "flex" the victim, that is, lift the victim with the rescuer's hands under his upper abdomen. This forces the water out. Squeeze the stomach, in the left upper quadrant of the abdomen, and/or squeeze the rib cage to force out any water in the lungs; follow this rapidly by standard CPR. Medical follow-up should be sought, since delayed metabolic effects commonly occur, especially in near-drowning in fresh water. These metabolic changes require intravenous administration of electrolytes (sodium, chloride, potassium) and require laboratory blood analyses.

Successful resuscitation from drownings or near-drownings has been reported after long periods of submersion in cold water (twenty to thirty minutes or more). This is especially true in children. Aggressive attempts should be made to begin and continue basic life support on near-drowning accidents.

HEART ATTACK

The heart is a muscle, and like all muscles, requires oxygen for metabolism. If the supply of oxygen to the heart muscle is diminished by the narrowing of its blood vessels, damage to the muscle cells can occur, which affects the ability of the heart muscle to contract, or to beat normally. This lack of blood supply causes *pain,* and the degree and duration of this pain generally reflects the seriousness of the heart's lack of oxygen.

Cardiac pain is typically located under the breastbone and is characterized as "tightness," "crushing," or "viselike" ("squeezing"). If it is severe and unrelenting, not affected by movement or breathing, radiates down the left arm, and is associated with sweating or nausea, it must be assumed to be a "coronary" (myocardial infarction) unless proved otherwise. High-risk individuals are overweight males who smoke and have high blood pressure or diabetes. (Any skipper you know?)

Therapy should involve immediate hospitalization. If this is not possible, the following should be done:

- Relieve pain (morphine sulfate subcutaneously, 2 to 15 mg).
- Put the victim at complete bed rest.
- Give oxygen if available—if not, plenty of fresh air.
- If possible give intravenous lidocaine to prevent rhythm abnormalities. Give 1 mg for every kilogram of the patient's weight. (1 kg = 2.2 lbs)

There is very little else that can be done on shipboard. If congestion develops in the victim's lungs, and breathing becomes noisy, rapid, and wet, a diuretic (Diuril, Lasix) may help.

HEAT ILLNESS

In 1841, aboard the British frigate *Liverpool* en route from Muscat to Bushire,

the weather gradually became warmer; double awnings were spread, the decks were kept constantly wetted and every precaution used to prevent exposure to the men. Yet in one day from species of coup de soleil, three lieutenants and thirty men were lost. It was stated at one time the decks resembled a slaughter house. . . .

Heat stroke (or "siriasis," based on a biblical reference to its occurrence with the appearance of the "dog star" Sirius, which could be seen in the twilight and followed the summer sun) is the most serious form of heat illness.

The heat-regulatory mechanisms of the body are extremely sensitive, so much so that fever is universally accepted as a hallmark of illness.

Metabolic heat in the body is eliminated by three means:

- By radiation to cooler surroundings.
- By convection by air coming in contact with the body.
- By evaporation, either from the surface of the skin through perspiration, or evaporation of moisture from the mucosal surfaces of the lungs and respiratory passages.

Any interference with these mechanisms will cause the body to retain heat. Existing atmospheric conditions influence these mechanisms. At 97° F and 30 percent humidity, no heat will be lost by radiation and convection, so that the main heat loss is by evaporation. If the temperature remains at 97° F and the humidity is raised to 100 percent saturation, all means of heat elimination fail, and sooner or later the body's sensitive thermostat will break down, causing a rise in body temperature, increasing respirations (to blow off heat) and increasing pulse rate. The metabolic rate also increases, which sets off a vicious cycle.

HEAT CRAMPS

Drinking water without replacing salt, while actively sweating, leads to painful muscle contractions. Temperature is normal. Salt depletion is present.

HEAT EXHAUSTION

This is probably an extension of heat cramps and is frequently seen in joggers. Symptoms are muscle cramps, profuse, drenching sweat, thirst, headache, dizziness, fainting or weakness, sometimes nausea and vomiting, rapid pulse rate, rapid respiration, lowered blood pressure, and a normal to slightly elevated temperature. It is caused by water depletion, salt depletion, or a combination of both, and the therapy is rehydration with salt-containing liquids—intravenously if necessary. Liberal salting of foods, salt tablets, cessation of activity, rest, and shade are preventative as well as therapeutic.

HEAT STROKE

This least common and most dangerous form of heat illness is characterized by very high body temperatures (greater than 105° F, 40° C) and the patient becomes delirious or comatose. The skin may be *dry,* meaning that the sweating mechanism has failed. Exercise or any other condition that increases the body's metabolic rate contributes to the syndrome—as do any factors that inhibit the body's ability to dissipate heat.

The primary goal of treatment is to lower the body's temperature *quickly.* A cool shady area, loose clothing (or none), immersion in a cold tub or cool ocean, or cold-water soaks with towels or sheets and vigorous fanning should be provided at once and continued *active* cooling should continue until the rectal temperature is 102° F or lower. Basic life support may be needed if the victim is comatose or has a convulsion because of the neurotoxic effects of the high body temperature. This is an emergency in every aspect, and medical help should be sought—although cooling the victim should not be postponed until it arrives. It should be noted that any condition, such as severe sunburn, which interferes with the sweating mechanism, can precipitate these heat illnesses.

CHAPTER 10

Prevention of Injuries at Sea

In each chapter of this book I have attempted to emphasize the prevention of each type of injury. Some general comments here relate to boating safety in general.

MAN OVERBOARD

It is hard for the neophyte sailor to envision how difficult it can be to retrieve a person who has fallen into the sea, especially in difficult weather conditions. And these are the very conditions that promote falling overboard. Prevention is by safety harness, attached to a fixed and solid portion of the boat, as well as stanchions, lifelines, and bow and stern pulpits. The techniques of recovery should be practiced beforehand so that every member of the crew is aware of the procedure. The simple act of throwing a life preserver overboard is frequently forgotten in the excitement when someone goes overboard. Proper flotation devices and a weighted float with a long "pick-up stick" may mean the difference between success or failure. The man-overboard drill is a must for all responsible skippers. The techniques are to be found in any sailing book worth its salt and I won't go into them here. Enough to say one must respect the forces one is dealing with.

Getting one's sea legs is an interesting phenomenon. I'm sure you are all aware of how awkward one can be the first day or so into a cruise and how agile one is at the end of a long passage. This adaptation to the motion of the boat, which is unconscious, takes time. Give yourself that time. Anticipate that awkwardness initially. Crawl, if you have to, on all fours. Foredeck work in a heavy sea can leave you airborne—even starting on all fours—so be prepared. Learn to work with one hand on the boat, the other at the job. If you need both hands, use a harness.

Nonskid deck paint, nonskid soles on your boat shoes, judicious use of water to rinse soapy decks after they've been washed, all help to improve the adhesion between man/woman and boat. I like bare feet, because they give me more tactile sensation and they are easier to dry than wet boat shoes. I admit it's a lot easier to stub one's toes that way—and probably to break them!!

BURNS/FIRES

Protection from the sun is a must as emphasized in Chapter 1. Sun block, a proper awning, a wide-brimmed hat, a long-sleeved shirt, especially early on in a sunny cruise, and a good pair of polarizing sunglasses are all essential.

Prevention is the name of the game for the dreaded engine or galley fire. Caution, a thorough knowledge of your stove and oven, and properly placed fire extinguishers are essential. Axioms regarding fuel fires are:

- Propane is invisible—and explosive.
- Alcohol is treacherous—and flammable.
- Gasoline fumes sink.
- "Listen to your nose in the engine room."

A pan of water should be readily available anytime alcohol is used for fuel. Alcohol is completely soluble in water and water is the most effective fire extinguisher for alcohol. When taking gasoline aboard, close all hatches below and use your blower before starting up. When boarding a boat that has been closed up for a time, smell the closed spaces, air out the boat, and blow out the engine compartment. Be afraid of fire on board. Burns are terrible injuries—to people and boats! When lighting propane stoves without pilot lights, light the match *before* the propane valve is opened. Also, shut off the main propane valve to extinguish the flame, thus letting it burn off.

Scalding burns occur all too commonly at sea. Heat uncovered liquids on calm days, at anchor or in harbor. Gimbaled or double gimbaled stoves are a must. The stove and oven should be positioned so that things don't continually pour or fall on the cook, on port or starboard tacks. A variety of "pot stoppers" exist on the market today and may save someone's getting burned or scalded by hot soup or hot grease in a pan. Do not overfill pots. Pressure cookers usually are quite handy in a boat's galley, and they are safe if used properly. No matter how beautiful your mate looks in a bikini, have her wear a long apron or slacks when at the galley. Burn scars are ugly and forever!

PREVENTIVE MAINTENANCE

Many injuries occur because things break, or loosen, and become missiles or free-falling objects. A daily "walk around and crawl under" type of inspection, like a preflight inspection of an airplane, would probably pick up potential problems, both structural and mechanical, *before* they occur and possibly cause injury. Check rigging, sheets, and shrouds. Simply laying a hand on a stay can give the skipper a feel for its tension or lack thereof. Check the engine oil, even if you don't use the engine all the time! Is there too much (any?) water in the bilge? Where is it coming from? Is there oil in the bilge? Is there gasoline or diesel fuel in the bilge? Checks of batteries, fuses, wires, electrical panels should be part of the day-to-day habits of a skipper on a cruise. When he gets to a point where he can "feel" something amiss, a skipper is "tuned in" to his boat. Don't compromise. Also, don't assume you can fix something that you are not familiar with. Anticipate things going wrong and plan for them. Have a spare-parts kit and replace items as they are used.

GEAR

Always use a "preventer" when off the wind. Fatigue, distraction, any momentary lack of concentration leading to an inadvertent jibe can potentially lead to a fatal head injury, not to mention disabling injury to the boat. Similarly, main-sheet tracks under great tension on the wind have been known to "let go," causing serious injury to whatever body part is in the path of this obvious weapon. Frayed lines, worn stays, or fractured stops don't deserve one's confidence. C. Waldo Howland, designer (along with Ray Hunt) of the classic Concordia yawls once told me that the more gear you add to your boat, the more can go wrong. Today's "modern" cruising yachts, with microwave ovens, electric refrigeration, air conditioning, diesel heaters, generators, electric "automatic" pumps, need a systems engineer to run them. In planning any cruise, anticipate that *everything is going to break,* and provide yourself with adequate, simple, backup systems, as well as the knowledge to accomplish your goals without these conveniences.

CHAPTER 11

Emergency Procedures

AIRWAY

Most airway problems will be controllable with a bag and a mask (AMBU). The technique involves positioning the patient's head so that there is no obstruction to the flow of air. This position involves advancing the chin outward ("jaw thrust") with the head and neck in the main plane of the body, not flexed or extended.

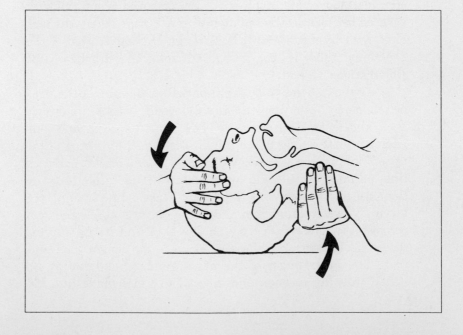

If properly positioned, with the airway cleared of debris, dentures, food (by sweeping the index finger across the mouth and throat), adequate ventilation at a rate of 10 to 15 breaths a minute can be maintained. Insertion of an oropharyngeal airway (through the mouth into the throat) may help. The airway should be inserted upside down and rotated 180° once positioned in the throat.

A *nasal* airway may also be used if there is injury to the mouth. This should be inserted *after clearing the mouth and throat* manually, as before, and is inserted with the natural curve leading through the nose into the throat.

If upper-airway obstruction cannot be relieved by these rather simple maneuvers, a *cricothyroidotomy* may have to be done. This is simpler and safer than a tracheotomy mainly because the cricothyroid membrane is close to the skin. This membrane is located in the mid-portion of the neck. If one runs a finger from the front of the chin downward toward the breastbone, the first "bump" the finger encounters is the Adam's apple—the upper edge of the thyroid cartilage. If one slides the finger over this prominence and continues downward the next bump is the cricoid cartilage and the depression just above this bump is the cricothyroid space, which is covered by the cricothyroid membrane. This is where the incision is to be made and it is through this space that a tracheotomy tube is to be passed into the trachea. (See illustrations 42 and 43.)

Again, it helps to be familiar with this area of the neck before doing your first cricothyroidotomy, so feel your own neck and learn it on yourself. The key to success and simplicity in performing this procedure is the stabilization of the upper part of the trachea with one's nondominant hand. If time permits, instill local anesthesia (1% lidocaine, ⅔ cc) in the skin and tissues over the space. Then, while holding the larynx between thumb and middle finger for stabilization, cut *transversely* (crosswise) through the skin and its underlying thin muscle layer. The incision need be no longer than one inch. The index finger of the nondominant hand can be inserted into the incision and direct the knife blade into the

42. Anatomy for Cricothyroidotomy
43. Technique of Cricothyroidotomy

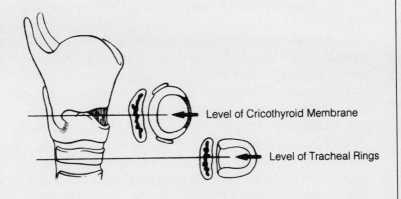

Level of Cricothyroid Membrane

Level of Tracheal Rings

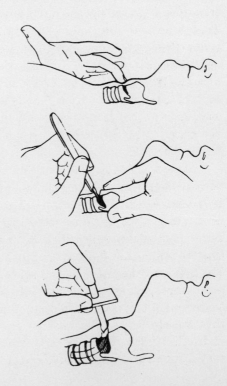

thin membrane, which is punctured with the knife blade held transversely. Turning the blade will enlarge the opening to allow the tip of the curved hemostat to be passed into it. One can enlarge the opening by spreading the jaws of the hemostat. Stay in the midline of the neck. Spread the opening and insert the tracheotomy tube so that it curves downward into the trachea.

Secure the tube in place with tape or use umbilical tape passed under the neck and tied to each side of the flange of the trach tube.

The tube itself can then be connected to the AMBU bag for positive control of ventilation.

The vast majority of airway problems should be able to be adequately handled with the measures described. These techniques, of course, vary from indirect (oral airway) to direct (cricothyroidotomy). The use of an endotracheal tube, which we have not described, is also quite direct but requires time and teaching for the novice and cannot be relied upon in an emergency situation unless the individual already had learned the skill. If indeed a skipper is experienced in placing an endotracheal tube, he should by all means pass it when airway obstruction exists.

CHEST TUBES

Insertion of a chest tube for pneumothorax has been alluded to previously. The techniques will be reviewed here.

After infiltration of the skin and subcutaneous tissue with local anesthetic in the area of the 5th interspace* (below the 5th rib), a small incision is made in line with the center of the armpit. This incision can be tunneled upward with the gloved finger feeling the ribs above and below and the chest wall beneath. The tube should be directed, similarly, upward

---

*The 5th interspace can be identified by counting the ribs from the top of the armpit downward. The highest rib is rib #1 (and it's way up there!) Even if the highest rib is missed, it is not a major error to use the 6th interspace.

44. Technique for Insertion of Chest Tube
45. Underwater Seal

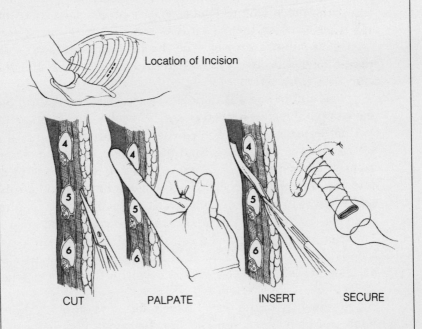

Location of Incision

CUT   PALPATE   INSERT   SECURE

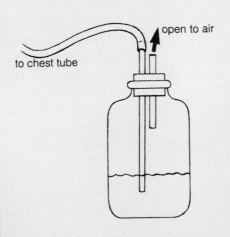

open to air

to chest tube

and inward—and if grasped with a curved clamp (Kelly, Carmalt) can be poked *into* the chest cavity, released, the clamp withdrawn, and the tube hooked up to a one-way valve (see Chapter X) or to an underwater seal. (See illustrations 44 and 45.)

This simple seal, as long as it is *below the patient's chest,* will allow air from the chest cavity out, and act as a one-way valve. The valve is simpler. The chest tube can be sutured in place—a stitch taken in the skin and then tied around the tube. (See illustration 44.)

The end of the tube should be clamped shut until the one-way valve or underwater seal is hooked up so that air will not enter the chest during the procedure.

If there is any oozing from the incision, the sutures will usually take care of it. A pressure dressing, cut to accommodate the exit of the tube, will also help. This should be securely taped in place.

GIVING AN INJECTION

Frequently in the text, I have referred to administration of medication by injection. The first step in giving an injection is to CHECK THE DOSAGE. The ampule may contain, for example, 10 milligrams of drug per milliliter or cubic centimeter. You may want to administer 5 mg. Simply stated:

$$\frac{\text{desired dose (mg)}}{\text{concentration in hand (mg/ml)}} = \text{ml to be given}$$

and in one example

$$\frac{5 \text{ mg}}{10 \text{ mg/ml}} = .5 \text{ ml to be given}$$

If the dose is ordered on the basis of weight—that is, milligrams per kilograms or pounds of body weight, remember that 1 kg equals 2.2 lbs., and that the average man weighs 70 kg (154 lbs.). It is a good idea to have a medical log on your crew: weight, allergies, current or past illnesses, especially if chronic (asthma, diabetes, hypertension, heart disease) as well as any drugs they are taking.

Most emergency drugs are currently available in prefilled syringes. This convenience prevents both wastage and contamination of multiple-dose vials. The shelf life is about the same as for multiple-dose vials if they are properly sealed and protected from the elements.

Subcutaneous Injection

1. Check dosage and check *label*.
2. Choose syringe with 25-gauge needle.
3. Select site for injection. The skin over the deltoid muscle in the upper arm is preferred.
4. Cleanse site with alcohol swab.
5. Pinch skin with thumb and forefinger, pulling it away from underlying muscle.
6. Insert needle at 45° angle to skin and administer dosage.
7. Withdraw needle and massage area.

Intramuscular Injection

1. Select 1½ inch needle with syringe appropriate for volume to be delivered.
2. The same site, or the upper outer quadrant of the gluteus, may be used.
3. Cleanse site with alcohol swab.
4. Instead of pinching skin, spread it out with thumb and index finger, stretching skin over the muscle.
5. Inject at 90° angle to the skin surface.
6. Withdraw and massage.

A little practice will help. As with all techniques in this section, rapid insertion of the needle is less painful. The selection of routes of drug administration depends on the rapidity with which the action of the drug is desired (or needed); subcutaneous injections are more slowly absorbed than intravenous injections. Drugs can also be administered under the tongue, by mouth, and rectally. Drugs given by the endotracheal route are very rapidly absorbed. The slowest rate of absorption is the oral route.

The intravenous route is rapid and accurately absorbed. However, the ability to administer drugs intravenously (or to start an I.V. line again) awaits advanced training. This training (advanced EMT or paramedic) would be very beneficial to any serious long-distance skipper, but it would be impractical for the majority.

Intravenous Insertion

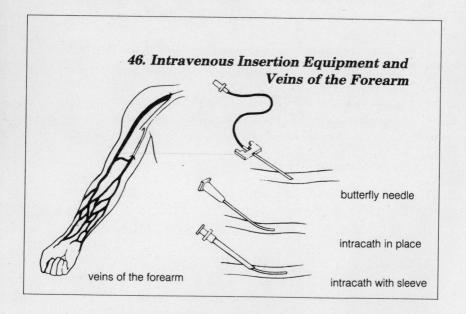

46. Intravenous Insertion Equipment and Veins of the Forearm

butterfly needle

intracath in place

veins of the forearm

intracath with sleeve

Preparation here is the key. Have all necessary equipment ready before puncturing the vein—that is, appropriate infusion bottle, administration set, proper syringe and needle, tape for securing the line if it is to be left in, a tourniquet.

A suitable vein is selected, usually by allowing

the arm to hang downward for a few minutes. Apply the tourniquet above the elbow in midarm, checking the pulse to make sure arterial *in*flow is not being obstructed. Look for a distended vein that is straight, and lay the arm on a relatively flat surface.

Stabilize the vein by applying pressure beyond the anticipated point of needle entry and prepare the area with iodine or alcohol. The needle must pass first through the skin and then into the vein. Point the bevel of the needle upward. There is a distinct feeling when the needle enters the vein and blood will return through the needle or into the syringe. If an I.V. line is to be started, secure the needle with adhesive strips after filling the entire system with the fluid to be administered. Make sure no air bubbles remain in the I.V. tubing and make sure there is no pull on the needle after the tubing is hooked up. This is best done by judicious use of adhesive strips.

Make sure that the fluid flow is steady, and that there is no swelling around the site of the needle entry, which would suggest that the fluid is *infiltrating* around the vein. If this is the case, remove the needle and start fresh.

In administering I.V. solutions, adjust the rate of flow to the time period over which it is to be given. Standard I.V. sets usually deliver 10 drops/cc.

CHAPTER 12

The "Ideal" Medical Kit

Throughout this book I have made reference to the "Ideal" Medical Kit. I have put together in this chapter all you will need in terms of drugs, bandages, splints, instruments, and other medical gear to minister to your crew. In some instances this kit will seem extravagant. It can be individualized for the extent of your cruising.

Airway Maintenance Equipment

AMBU mask and bag
Oxygen—portable tanks
Suctioning equipment—bulb syringe
Airways (oral)—sizes 5 and 6 (children)
　　　　　　　—sizes 2 and 3 (children)
Laryngoscope and endotracheal tubes

Cricothyroidotomy Equipment

Scalpel
#15 blades
Hemostats, curved
Tracheotomy tube—#6/#8 with cuff

Tubing

Chest tubes—#24, #28 (Argyll)
Rubber gloves or condoms for one-way flap valve

Nasogastric tubes—#16 Diagram 41
Foley catheters—#16, #5 cc bag Diagram 40

Syringes

Sterile disposable syringes—2½/6 cap
25/21 gauge needles
Large-bore needles—12 gauge/14 gauge
Bulb syringes—large volume (Davol)

Bandages/Splints

4 × 4 gauze pads
Adaptic—2"/3"/4"
Kling—2"/3"/4"
Ace—2"/3"/4"
Steristrips—small, medium, large
Tape—adhesive, cloth, plastic
Air splints—1 set (long leg, long arm)
Universal hand splint
Vaseline gauze
Eye patches (1 doz.)
Q-Tips
Slings or material (muslin) for same

General Supplies

Clorox
Salt
Vinegar
Ammonia
Adolph's meat tenderizer
Aloe
Peroxide, 3%
Cold packs
K-Y jelly
Vaseline

Anesthetic Agents (Local)

Marcaine without epinephrine, .5%
Tetracaine ophthalmic, .5%
Xylocaine gel, 2%

Antibiotics

Systemic—General
Penicillin G, 400,000 U/tablet
Tetracycline 250 mg tablets
Cephalothin 500 mg tablets

Systemic—Urinary
Gantrisin 0.5 mg tablets
Septra tablets

Topical
Silvadene—20 mg tubes
Bacitracin ointment
Neosporin powder—15 gm bottles
Chloromycetin Ophthalmic, 1%
Betadine/Clinidine salve

Antispasmodics/Antiemetics

Atropine—0.1 ml/5 ml syringe (Abbott)
Banthine—50 mg tablets
Valium—5 mg tablets
Transderm-Scōp (scopolamine)

Antihistamines

Benadryl—25/50 mg capsules

Antiseptics

Betadine plus scrub brushes
Peroxide, 3%
pHisoHex
Clinidine salve

Soporifics

Valium—5 mg tablets
Phenobarbital—100 mg tablets

Analgesics

For moderate pain: Demerol 100 mg tablets
For severe pain   : Morphine Tubex (Wyeth) 10 milli-
                   grams per c.c.
For mild pain   : Tylenol with codeine capsules
                   Aspirin #4

Emergency Cardiac Drugs

Lidocaine, 1%
Epinephrine Tubex (Wyeth), 1:1,000
Calcium gluconate—Dosette syringes, 1 gm/10 ml
(Elkins-Sinn, Inc.)
Sodium bicarbonate—Bristoject syringes (Bristol), 50
mg/50 ml

Steroids

Kenalog ointment
Prednisone—5 mg tablets

Miscellaneous

Tincture of benzoin for adhesion
Foam-rubber padding

Surgical Instruments

1 Needle holder
Scissors
Bandages
Sutures
Forceps—2 pair toothed, plain
Hemostats—curved

Prepackaged suture material

4-0 Nylon on cutting needle (Ethilon)

Emetics

Syrup of ipecac
Activated charcoal granules

Special Equipment

Antivenin (See Chapter II)
I.V. administration sets
5% Dextrose/saline—in plastic bags
Tourniquet
Blood pressure cuff and gauge
Thermometer
Stethoscope

It is possible to obtain many of these medications in "dosepaks." This saves a lot of figuring of volumes and, with infrequent use, will probably save expense. Sterile *disposable* materials should be purchased where possible. The packaging of these products for sea presents very special problems. Ziploc bags are extremely important, as is a heavy-duty plastic case to hold everything, which itself can be sealed with enough air inside to allow it to float.